T0202408

The Ethics of Shared Decision Making

The Ethics of Shared Decision Making

Edited by

JOHN D. LANTOS, MD

Professor
Department of Pediatrics
Children's Mercy Hospital and University of Missouri
Kansas City, MO, USA

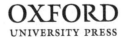

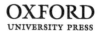

Oxford University Press is a department of the University of Oxford. It furthers
the University's objective of excellence in research, scholarship, and education
by publishing worldwide. Oxford is a registered trade mark of Oxford University
Press in the UK and certain other countries.

Published in the United States of America by Oxford University Press
198 Madison Avenue, New York, NY 10016, United States of America.

Library of Congress Cataloging-in-Publication Data
Names: Lantos, John D., editor.
Title: The ethics of shared decision making / John D. Lantos, editor.
Description: New York, NY : Oxford University Press, [2021] |
Includes bibliographical references and index.
Identifiers: LCCN 2021008098 (print) | LCCN 2021008099 (ebook)
ISBN 9780197598573 (hardback) | ISBN 9780197598597 (epub) |
ISBN 9780197598603 (online)
Subjects: MESH: Clinical Decision-Making—ethics |
Decision Making, Shared | Physician-Patient Relations—ethics |
Patient Rights—ethics
Classification: LCC R724 (print) | LCC R724 (ebook) | NLM WB 142.5 |
DDC 174.2—dc23
LC record available at https://lccn.loc.gov/2021008098
LC ebook record available at https://lccn.loc.gov/2021008099

DOI: 10.1093/med/9780197598573.001.0001

This material is not intended to be, and should not be considered, a substitute for medical or other
professional advice. Treatment for the conditions described in this material is highly dependent on the
individual circumstances. And, while this material is designed to offer accurate information with respect
to the subject matter covered and to be current as of the time it was written, research and knowledge about
medical and health issues are constantly evolving and dose schedules for medications are being revised
continually, with new side effects recognized and accounted for regularly. Readers must therefore always
check the product information and clinical procedures with the most up-to-date published product
information and data sheets provided by the manufacturers and the most recent codes of conduct and
safety regulations. The publisher and the authors make no representations or warranties to readers,
express or implied, as to the accuracy or completeness of this material. Without limiting the foregoing, the
publisher and the authors make no representations or warranties as to the accuracy or efficacy of the drug
dosages mentioned in the material. The authors and the publisher do not accept, and expressly disclaim,
any responsibility for any liability, loss, or risk that may be claimed or incurred as a consequence of the use
and/or application of any of the contents of this material.

3 5 7 9 8 6 4 2

Printed by Integrated Books International, United States of America

Contents

Contributors

Jennifer Blumenthal-Barby, PhD, MA
Cullen Professor of Medical Ethics and Associate Director
Center for Medical Ethics and Health Policy
Baylor College of Medicine
Houston, TX, USA

Daniel Brudney, PhD
Professor
Department of Philosophy
The University of Chicago
Chicago, IL, USA

Jonna D. Clark, MD, MA
Pediatric Critical Care Physician; Associate Professor
Pediatric Critical Care;
Department of Pediatrics
Seattle Children's Hospital, University of Washington
Seattle, WA, USA

Melissa K. Cousino, PhD
Associate Professor
Department of Pediatrics
University of Michigan
Ann Arbor, MI, USA

Sabrina F. Derrington, MD, MA, HEC-C, FAAP
Director of the CHLA Center for Pediatric Bioethics; Associate Professor of Clinical Pediatrics
Department of Anesthesiology and Critical Care Medicine
Children's Hospital Los Angeles; Keck School of Medicine of the University of Southern California
Los Angeles, CA, USA

Chris Feudtner, MD, PhD, MPH
Professor of Pediatrics, Medical Ethics and Health Policy
Steven D. Handler Endowed Chair of Medical Ethics
Director of the Department of Medical Ethics
Children's Hospital of Philadelphia
Philadelphia, PA, USA

Alexander G. Fiks, MD, MSCE
Associate Professor of Pediatrics, Director of the Center for Pediatric Clinical Effectiveness
Department of Pediatrics
Children's Hospital of Philadelphia
Philadelphia, PA, USA

Jodi Halpern, MD, PhD
Professor of Bioethics
UCB-UCSF Joint Medical Program
and School of Public Health
University of California
Berkeley, CA, USA

Douglas L. Hill, PhD
Social Psychologist
Justin Michael Ingerman Center
for Palliative Care
The Children's Hospital of
Philadelphia
Philadelphia, PA, USA

Alexander A. Kon, MD, HEC-C,
FAAP, FCCM
Clinical Professor
Department of Pediatrics and
Bioethics
University of Washington School
of Medicine
Seattle, WA, USA
Clinical Professor
Department of Pediatrics
University of California San Diego
School of Medicine
San Diego, CA, USA

John D. Lantos, MD
Professor
Department of Pediatrics
Children's Mercy Hospital and
University of Missouri
Kansas City, MO, USA

Mithya Lewis-Newby, MD, MPH
Associate Professor, Divisions of
Pediatric Critical Care Medicine
and Bioethics/Palliative Care
Department of Pediatrics
Seattle Children's Hospital,
University of Washington School
of Medicine
Seattle WA, USA

Victoria A. Miller, PhD
Associate Professor and Pediatric
Psychologist
Department of Pediatrics
Children's Hospital of Philadelphia
Philadelphia, PA, USA

Wynne Morrison, MD, MBE
Professor
Anesthesiology and Critical Care
Perelman School of Medicine at
the University of Pennsylvania
and the Children's Hospital of
Philadelphia
Philadelpha PA, USA

Douglas J. Opel, MD, MPH
Associate Professor
Department of Pediatrics
University of Washington School
of Medicine; Treuman Katz
Center for Pediatric Bioethics,
Seattle Children's Research
Institute
Seattle, WA, USA

Aleksa Owen, PhD, MSW
Evaluation and Practice Fellow
National Center on Disability in
    Public Health
Association of University Centers
    on Disabilities
Silver Spring, MD, USA

Erin Paquette, MD, JD, MBe
Assistant Professor
Pediatrics (Critical Care) and
    School of Law (by courtesy)
Northwestern University Feinberg
    School of Medicine and Pritzker
    School of Law (by courtesy)
Chicago, IL, USA

Kimberly E. Sawyer, MD, MA
Assistant Member
Department of Oncology
St. Jude Children's Research
    Hospital
Memphis, TN, USA

Theodore E. Schall, MSW, MBE
PhD Student
Department of Health Policy and
    Management
Johns Hopkins School of
    Public Health
Baltimore, MD, USA

Mark Siegler, MD, MACP
Lindy Bergman Distinguished
    Service Professor of Medicine
    and Surgery, Founding Director
    (1984)of the MacLean Center
    of Clinical Medical Ethics,
Executive Director, The
    Bucksbaum Institute for Clinical
    Excellence
Medicine (section of General
    Internal Medicine)
The University of Chicago
Chicago, IL, USA

Jennifer K. Walter, MD, PhD, MS
Associate Professor of Pediatrics
    and Medical Ethics
Department of Pediatrics
University of Pennsylvania School
    of Medicine
Philadelphia, PA, USA

1

Introduction

The Fascinating Synergy of Shared Decision Making

John D. Lantos

There are some paradoxes in the way doctors and patients make medical decisions today. Today's patients are more empowered than were patients in the past. They have the right to see their medical records. The law requires doctors to obtain their informed consent for treatment. Patients are told about the options for treatment and the risks and benefits of each option. Their values and preferences are elucidated to guide the treatments that are provided.

As a result of these processes, and through the democratization of medical information, patients are more knowledgeable today than they have ever been before. They have access to peer-reviewed medical journals. Medical articles are extensively covered in the lay press. Social media allows patients to share stories with other patients and to learn about other people's experiences with various treatments. There are websites for patients written by experts at leading medical schools. But different websites may give very different advice or may avoid giving advice at all.

The contradictory nature of publicly available information is inevitable and likely to increase. Medical progress takes place unevenly. Innovative treatments have unknown risks and benefits. Doctors often disagree with each other and with administrators or policymakers. With so much information available, it is hard to know what to trust. Thus, although patients have more access to medical information today than they ever did before, they may also be more confused and in need of guidance. Patients may thus turn to a trusted physician to guide them through the dense thicket of conflicting information, incompatible recommendations, and risky choices. They don't want doctors to make decisions, but they need doctors' help to make decisions themselves.

Doctors today have a role that is also quite different from the role they had in the past. They no longer dictate treatment. Instead, doctors need to provide each patient with the information the patient needs to make the treatment decisions that are best. There is no single right answer. Today, doctors have much more knowledge about the safety and efficacy of treatments than doctors had in the past. They know more thanks to learning health care systems and rigorous comparative effectiveness studies. The decision making gets more complex as innovative treatments compete with established ones, as genomic information allows for highly personalized assessment of the risks and benefits of different treatment options, and as health insurance coverage may lead to vastly different out-of-pocket costs associated with different treatment choices.

The implications of all these changes are clear. Doctors and patients need to help one another. It is a partnership that can be uncomfortable for both. Some patients want an old-fashioned doctor who will tell them what to do. Others want to be in charge of their own decisions but need help and guidance to exercise their autonomy. Doctors need to be nimble in figuring out what role each patient wants to play and, as a result, what role the doctor must play to help them. All of this takes place against the historical background of traditional roles for doctors and patients, roles that are still comfortable for many people. The implicit shifts in roles are usually not explicitly discussed. Furthermore, the decisions that must be made are emotionally fraught. Patients are often trying to make decisions just as they've been told that they have a life-threatening illness. Treatment choices often have life-altering consequences. There is often time pressure to make a decision quickly. Family members may be involved and may be helpful or detrimental to the patient's emotional well-being.

These paradoxes have led to an interesting and incompletely theorized new approach to medical decision making. Doctors and patients work together today to make the many decisions that are necessary in both acute and chronic illnesses. This approach has been labeled "shared decision making" (SDM) and is thought to be a middle ground between pure paternalism and unbridled autonomy.

SDM sounds good in theory. In practice, however, it can be quite complex. Doctors sometimes need to be directive and to make a recommendation. At other times, they need to strive for neutrality. It is not always clear which approach is most appropriate for which situations, even as both doctor and patient have the same goal—to get to the overall best outcomes for the patient. The conversations and decisional negotiations may turn on an attempt to figure out what, exactly, each means by the word "best."

The demise of paternalism was due primarily to confusion over what is best. Doctors may think that survival is always best, but patients may be more concerned about their quality of life. Alternatively, doctors may think that some side effects of treatment would be intolerable, while patients may be willing to live with those side effects. Often, patients have more than one health problem and there is more than one treatment for each of their health problems. Treatment for one may exacerbate another. Choices, then, cannot simply be based on empirical scientific evidence. They must also reflect the patient's values and priorities. There are, often, a number of different medically reasonable options. Some of these options will be more appealing to some patients than others.

The physician, then, has the complex role of helping the patient understand the choices and make the best one in light of their own values. Physicians must offer their expertise in a way that guides the patient but does so without being overly directive. This is a tricky communicative task. It requires careful listening, thoughtful choice of words, awareness of one's own biases, sensitivity to the patient's needs, and a cautious calibration of directiveness. The task is very different from the task of trying to provide information in a value-neutral way. The nature of the physician's role and goals is such that it is seldom desirable, or possible, to be completely neutral. Physicians may have deeply held beliefs about what is best for each particular patient at each particular decision point. But physicians need to be aware of their own values and must decide when to advocate for those values and when to defer to the patient's values. With awareness of one's own goals and biases, one can also be more aware of the way one frames choices.

Clinicians are trained to know which treatments have which probability of leading to which outcome. Patients specify the goals or outcomes they wish to achieve. Clinicians are wiser about the efficacy of various treatments but are *not* wiser about appropriate goals. Thus, the clinician must use practical wisdom to facilitate the patient's understanding of their values and goals so that the patient can be in a position to evaluate the options before them.

The process of SDM is complex and nuanced and requires a delicate balance of power between doctor and patient. In many cases, it requires input from many doctors and not just the patient but also the patient's loved ones. It is an ongoing and open-ended process that, in the context of ongoing medical care, usually requires not one decision but many different decisions, over time, in the context of continuously changing clinical situations. At its best, it leads to a fascinating synergy between doctor and patient through which each party's input is considered and creates a holistic understanding that is greater than the sum of its parts.

The goal of this book is to offer different perspectives on the process of SDM to help health professionals and patients understand the process and do it better.

Chris Feudtner; Theodore Schall; and Douglas Hill show that decisions evolve over the course of an illness and that doctors and patients (or their surrogates) must make decisions in a way that is consistent with their own ideas about their proper roles. Doctors understand the many ways that they must aspire to be "good doctors." But, in a similar way, surrogate decision makers must try to understand the moral demands that go along with their role. Like doctors, they too have duties and obligations that must be honored.

Mark Siegler gives a brief history of the ways that the doctor-patient relationship changed in the last half of the 20th century. He then outlines the process by which clinicians and patients negotiate the terms of their collaboration. It begins with the patient's recognition that they need expert guidance, progresses to the clinician's evaluation of options, and concludes with a negotiated decision about how the two will work together.

Daniel Brudney delves more deeply into the philosophical reasons that physician paternalism is on the decline but also patients still turn to physicians to seek their practical wisdom and guidance as they consider treatment options.

Jodi Halpern and Aleksa Owen show some of the ways that physicians can inadvertently shape decisions when physicians, unaware of their own biases about particular treatments, frame decisions in such a way that leads patients to make choices that may not be the best in the circumstances.

Jonna Clark; Mithya Lewis-Newby; Alexander A. Kon; and Wynne Morrison introduce the concept of titrated directiveness in their discussion of the broad spectrum of approaches that are available to physicians as they partner with patients.

Jennifer Walter and Alexander Fiks discuss different conceptual models for SDM and provide practical guidance about the ways that physicians can improve their communication skills. They conclude that, in spite of many well-described models, there is limited practical guidance for physicians on how they should communicate with patients and their parents to achieve the goal of SDM. This chapter provides practical guidance.

Victoria Miller and Melissa Cousino try to tease out the modifications that are necessary if we are to use an SDM approach in children.

Kimberly Sawyer and Douglas J. Opel present a practical 4-step framework for SDM. After the physician explains the medically reasonable options along with the benefits and burdens of each, the patient and physician then evaluate each option in light of the patient's values and the anticipated outcomes.

Sabrina Derrington and Erin Paquette offer a closer look at the concept of culture as it relates to communication and decision making. Specific recommendations are provided to improve cross-cultural communication to optimize the process of shared decision making.

Jennifer Blumenthal-Barby analyzes the impact of the biases and heuristics that both clinicians and patients use to arrive at decisions. It shows how these influence autonomy by shaping people's understanding and their intentionality in making choices that reflect their values.

Finally, John D. Lantos talks about the meaning of truth telling in the context of SDM. He discusses the different ways that clinicians can choose to tell the truth and the ways that patients or their surrogates communicate their values.

2

Surrogate's Personal Sense of Duty as a Crucial Element in Medical Decision Making

Ethical, Empirical, and Experience-Based Perspectives

Chris Feudtner, Theodore E. Schall, and Douglas L. Hill

Prologue

The small, windowless room was down at the end of a hallway in the NICU. The pair of doctors entered ahead of us, followed by the bedside nurse, as the social worker held open the door for us to all file in. My partner and I knew all these people. They were nice; they had been taking care of my 4-month-old daughter for her entire life. We knew how sick she was, about the brain bleed that she had that first week of life, and now how bad her lungs were. And we knew that we were going to talk about whether or not we should move ahead with a tracheostomy. But as we sat down, I kept wondering—as I had for weeks and weeks—how a parent could even begin to think about this kind of decision.

When we have to make decisions for others—perhaps as a parent deciding for a child, or an adult child deciding for an aged parent—how do we approach not only the specific task of making a particular decision but also the encompassing task of being a surrogate decision maker?[1,2]

Many discussions of shared decision making focus on the first, more specific task. We believe that the second task is far more important. Our main thesis is that specific decisions are shaped by individuals' personal understanding of the role of the surrogate decision maker. Whoever is entrusted or authorized to make medical decisions for another person, that decision maker operates within the framework of a personal sense of duty and an understanding of the major responsibilities of being a good surrogate decision maker. This person adopts particular beliefs or devises specific rules that they believe a "good" surrogate decision maker should follow. When support for surrogate decision makers focuses too much on the details of medical intervention options and not enough on assisting with the confusions, dilemmas, and self-recriminations inherent in trying to formulate a guiding personal duty to serve in the role of surrogate decision maker, the process is doomed to fail.

Our understanding derives from clinical experience, from personal experience as a surrogate decision maker, and from studies of clinical decision making and more general behavioral research. We have done such studies with parents of children with serious illness. We have also been clinicians providing complex and palliative care to children and young adults. We have cared for dying parents.

Our view is a commonsense view. Decision making is typically not a single, instantaneous event. Rather, decision making plays out and evolves over time. The ways in which decision making plays out, the relationships that develop, and the context in which decisions are made all provide both the framework and the constraints for decisions.

We present the remainder of our hypothetical case in the form of a multiact play, complete with an epilogue, and after each part we address specific assumptions embedded in how ethicists and decision-support advocates conceptualize what are—we wish to emphasize—the separate but paired tasks of making shared medical decisions and making medical decisions for someone else.

Obscured by Simplicity: Assumption of a Clear and Set Problem Structure

The attending described again the many problems with our daughter's lungs. She recalled the various discussions that we'd had along the way. She had a long agenda for the meeting: she wanted to talk about what a tracheostomy was and what going home someday on a ventilator might look like, and to go through the pros and cons of doing this. She also wanted to talk about what would happen if we did not move forward with the tracheostomy and instead focused on our daughter's comfort, knowing that she would not live long that way. All I kept thinking was that there was no decision here—her bad lungs threatened her survival, and the tracheostomy was the only option.

In the half-century since the rise of informed consent in medical practice, the practice of clinicians sitting with patients or surrogate decision makers and outlining the medical problem, followed by a description of treatment options and their advantages and disadvantages, has become a well-worn routine, even if done, as often as not, inconsistently or poorly.[3-6] Embedded in this practice, though, is a key assumption that warrants attention.

The basic model of informed consent imagines a situation in which a patient has a single medical problem with several possible solutions. The patient or surrogate must choose among the possible options. This "one-to-many" model (see upper panel of Figure 2.1) structures the problematic situation and tries to reduce the complexity of the overall situation. This basic model presumes, and thereby essentially dictates, both "the" decision that has to be made

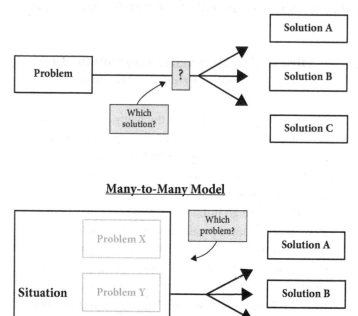

Figure 2.1 One-to-Many and Many-to-Many models of medical decision-making

and the range of possible choices. Importantly, although surrogate decision makers and clinicians often do not identify the same set of problems for a given patient,[7,8] the problem at hand is typically selected by the clinician.

The assumptions behind many models of shared decision making incorporate this basic one-to-many model. This leads to a goal of helping decision makers choose among the predefined possible solutions. Clinicians work with the patient or surrogate to clarify their values and preferences in ways that would help them choose among the potential solutions.[9,10] Depending upon patients' or surrogates' preferences about decision making, the clinician may have a larger or smaller role in recommending a particular treatment option.[11] This one-to-many model is the basic situation for which quantitative decision aids were designed. They help a patient understand what is at stake in a particular decision about a small number of choices.[12]

This basic model simplifies the complex reality of high-stakes medical decisions. Let's examine three aspects of this simplification. First, most serious medical conditions present several potential problems to the patient or the surrogate (see bottom panel of Figure 2.1). In a "many-to-many" model of decision making, the solution-oriented right side of the model is balanced by the problem-defining left side. Astute clinicians, who understand this, must spend much more effort defining and prioritizing the various problems that the patient and family face. Only then can they turn their attention to solving them. Defining the problem may not only enhance the quality of subsequent decisions (judged within the informed consent standard) but also improve long-term outcomes by enhancing adherence to treatment plans or minimizing decisional regret for both patients and surrogates.[13,14] Given these potential benefits, this more balanced clinical practice should be codified conceptually: ethicists and decision-making experts should not consider a complex of affiliated or linked problems as extraneous or irrelevant factors intruding inappropriately upon decision making, but instead view them as part of the fabric of decision making. Although this process is not explicitly within the scope of the basic model of informed consent, good clinicians and advocates of shared decision making have always understood the importance of defining the problems as part of values and preferences clarification.[9,10]

A second way that the one-to-many model oversimplifies the challenges of medical decision making is by depicting the making of "a" decision as a discrete act. This act of decision making may be time-consuming and complex. Decision making may take hours or days to complete. But once "the" decision has been made, formal ethical attention or decision support starts to fade. In ethics case discussions, the story of "what happened after the decision was made" is generally presented more or less as an informative coda. From the vantage of a patient with a serious illness or their surrogate decision maker, however, decision making is ongoing and continuous. Each decision leads to new situations that also require decisions. Like someone cast suddenly into a labyrinth, walking in search of a path that leads them out, the surrogate decision maker must choose again and again which way to turn (see Figure 2.2).

Third, in the setting of serious illness, the process of shared decision making between surrogate decision maker and clinician often takes more time than suggested by the basic one-to-many model. In practice, we believe that most critical care or complex care clinicians already know this to be the case. Importantly, though, because the processes of defining the problem and of making several decisions occur in series, clinicians can devote the required time not just to one big meeting but, more ideally, to a series of conversations about the ongoing decisions.

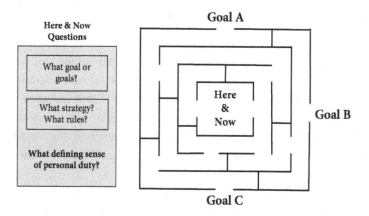

Figure 2.2 Labyrinthian model of medical decision-making

Inside a Labyrinth: Assumption of a Clear Approach to Medical Decision Making

As the attending started to talk about the tracheostomy, I felt the now-too-familiar sense of uncertainty and dread that had swept over me in prior conversations about what to do. Hardly a week had gone by when we hadn't needed to meet to discuss some bad news and what could be done. How had we gotten to this point? I knew we had come to a great hospital, but was this the best place for our daughter given how ill she had remained? Should we have pushed for a transfer to another hospital? Should we get a second opinion? Yet I had put my trust in these doctors, and they seemed really good. Everyone I talked to back home was supportive, but no one understood what we were going through. The day she was born so premature, our world had been turned upside down, and every week it seemed to flip over again. My head was spinning, but I needed to be strong and make a decision. But how could I live with myself if we didn't go for the tracheostomy?

The fact that patients and surrogates encounter repeated decision points in the care of the seriously ill patient is worthy of ethical attention.[15] The labyrinth metaphor suggests aspects of an illness journey that reflects that experience of complete disorientation that is reported by many parents and surrogate decision makers who confront a medical crisis for the first time. They can't see their way to a goal and thus see no clear, direct path forward. Instead, they feel lost, helpless, dependent, and confused. They cannot comprehend what is going on.[16-19]

Devotees of a basic model of informed consent or decision support might respond to a patient or parent's lack of comprehension by redoubling their efforts to explain what is going on by giving details of the medical condition and the pros and cons of proposed treatments. Patients or their loved ones are often hoping for the loved one's full recovery or, at least, their return to a previous baseline level of health. Some treatment decisions seem obviously related to that goal. For others, though, the relationship to the goal is less clear. Some treatments result in unexpected negative side effects. Such developments may seem like wrong choices or dead ends that lead the surrogate and the patient further into the labyrinth and away from their goal.

The metaphor of the labyrinth also captures the path dependency of medical decision making: past decisions influence present decisions. Over the course of time, decisions made earlier, such as what hospital to go to or what initial treatments to try, shape the way that surrogates approach later decisions as well as the decisions they have to make immediately. Parents of children with serious illness often say that the biggest decision they made was to come to our hospital. Once there, they were ready to trust our expertise and be told what was the best thing to do. For these parents, the decision of who to trust shaped all subsequent decisions. If later the parents learn that their child might benefit from a very specific treatment only offered at another institution, they may feel trapped by their past decision to go with the current hospital. Path dependence suggests that surrogates' decisions (both what they must decide and how they make the decision) are predicated upon the choices they made earlier. Reassessments and revisions of the medical plan, although based on the best information available at each decision point, may leave surrogates feeling more trapped and hopeless as they fail to make progress toward the goal of the patient's recovery.

These feelings are not just about what is going on with the patient. They also arise from the surrogates' thoughts about the role that they themselves should play.[19,20] The decisions that surrogates confront are about both the patient and themselves. They judge their own motives and actions, judgments that lead to decisions about who they are and what they will become.

From Roles to Rules: Assumption That Social Relationships Are Irrelevant

When the attending had finished educating us about tracheostomies and home ventilators, she then shifted to talk about how much our daughter had already suffered. She gently described to us what a "compassionate extubation" would be like. She and the social worker reassured us that we did not need to make any decision now. They just wanted to start preparing us for this decision. Then my partner asked: How have other parents made this type of decision? How will we know when too much is too much?

In the basic models of informed consent and medical decision support (operating within the framework of either substituted judgment or the best interests standard), the values and preferences of the patient or surrogate are clarified so that they can be applied to the work of evaluating treatment options, mostly in terms of the short- and long-term potential health benefits and risks. This approach assumes that each surrogate has a stable set of values and preferences that can be drawn out and applied to the decision. By this model, these values and preferences are independent of the surrogate's social roles or relationships with the patient and others. In other words, the same values could be applied to a decision for a sick parent, spouse, or child. We suggest that this is not the case for most decisions. The relationships between the surrogate decision maker and the patient are morally fundamental and shape the entire process of medical decision making.

Individuals' identities grow out of their well roles as professionals, spouses, parents, or friends. These roles give life meaning, purpose, and structure.[21,22] In these roles, people have specific rules or duties (see Figure 2.3). Spouses and adult children have different roles than do parents.[19,23,24] The role of "parent"

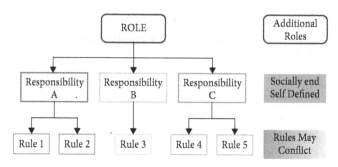

Figure 2.3 Roles, Responsibilities, and Rules

comes preloaded by social convention with a set of responsibilities and duties such as meeting basic needs, providing safety, keeping the child healthy and free from harm, and assisting with development.[25]

Over the past decade, we have worked to better understand how parents of ill children perceive their personal sense of duty. Much of this work has focused on improving our understanding of parental beliefs about what they, as a parent, should be most focused on for their child.[26] A range of beliefs have emerged (see Box 2.1), though not all parents hold the same beliefs with the same strength.[27,28] Beliefs are translated into action by "explicit heuristics," that is, by decision-making rules that facilitate or shape the performance of different tasks that are bound up in the role of being a parent of a child with a serious illness (see Table 2.1).[29] For any given parent, a set of good-parent beliefs combined with a set of explicit heuristics (as well as some unstated rules) allow parents to form their personal sense of duty.

This sense of duty serves as an overarching framework when making decisions (see Figure 2.4). A personal sense of duty provides a focus and orientation when trying to comprehend complex medical situations and sort through treatment options. Heuristics—be they explicit or implicit—enable judgments to be made about specific options. When parents or other surrogates undertake the task

Box 2.1 Examples of Good-Parent Beliefs

- Making sure my child feels loved
- Focusing on child's health
- Making informed medical care decisions
- Advocating for my child with medical staff
- Focusing on my child's comfort
- Focusing on my child's quality of life
- Putting my child's needs above my own when making medical care decisions
- Staying at my child's side
- Keeping a positive outlook
- Focusing on my child having as long a life as possible
- Focusing on my child's spiritual well-being
- Keeping a realistic outlook
- Doing right by my child
- Maintaining faith
- Having a legacy
- Being a good life example
- Letting the lord lead
- Making my child healthy
- Making sure my child feels loved
- Focusing on child's health
- Making informed medical care decisions
- Advocating for my child with medical staff
- Focusing on my child's comfort
- Focusing on my child's quality of life
- Putting my child's needs above my own when making medical care decisions
- Staying at my child's side
- Keeping a positive outlook
- Focusing on my child having as long a life as possible
- Focusing on my child's spiritual well-being

- Keeping a realistic outlook
- Doing right by my child
- Maintaining faith
- Having a legacy
- Being a good life example
- Letting the lord lead
- Making my child healthy

From Hinds et al.,[26] October et al.,[27] and Renjilian et al.[29]

Table 2.1 Explicit Heuristics

Purpose or Function	Examples
To depict or facilitate understanding of complex situations	• I just play it over and over again that our son's going to die. • This is my child. • Everything works for the good. • God is in control.
To clarify, organize, and focus pertinent information and values	• Take things day by day. • That's not even a decision. • Distinction between quality of days versus quantity of days. • I have to fight.
To serve as a decision-making compass, highlighting primary rule(s) to follow when making a decision	• We said we wanted them to do everything they can to keep our child alive. • I don't want my child to be in pain. • We just want her to be comfortable.
To communicate about a complex topic with others, including clinicians or family members	• There are no answers. There are never any answers. But he's sick. • We have to think outside of the box.
To justify a choice	• It was best for him. • It's not that we're giving up on her. • We've done everything in our power.

From Renjilian et al.[29]

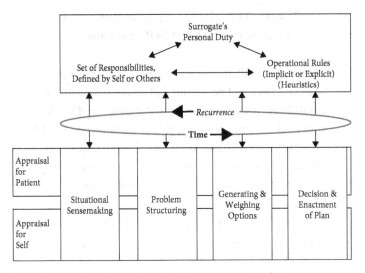

Figure 2.4 A More Complete Decision Support Model

of weighing options in light of their preferences and values, much of this weighing occurs by applying the heuristics derived from the rules that they have formulated based on their idea of what is required of them as the good parent, the good son, the loyal wife, the reliable older brother, and so on.

The search for a treatment to pursue is preceded by a search for and selection of a set of rules to follow. Surrogate decision makers may struggle to honor and fulfill their personally identified duties while also engaging in the shared decision-making process: the seemingly firm dictates of some of the explicit heuristics, such as that "we must not stop fighting," are at odds with the cognitive flexibility that the shared decision-making process requires.

Whispers in the Dark: Assumption of
Decisions Without Self-Judgments

> They had all left the room. We had asked for time to be alone. They had been kind and empathetic—they really did care about our daughter and about us. They had answered all our questions. While we knew we would never fully understand what either choice would entail, we felt that we had plenty of information. We sat in silence for a while. I was so upset, but so grateful that we were there together; I couldn't imagine doing this on my own. Then my partner said: "I don't want to be selfish." And I blurted out: "I'm going to feel so guilty, no matter what."

In reaching decisions, surrogates must listen to their own internal monologues. These focus on the decision that they face but are often framed in terms of their self-identity as a good parent. In these monologues, self-judgment can be lurking everywhere.[30,31]

To advance decision support, we need to appreciate the role that these inner deliberations have on the decision-making process. Surrogate decision makers make fundamental moralistic judgments about what they must do to be good or which choices would lead to a self-perception that they are bad. When individuals fall short of their desired self-identity, they experience depression and anxiety.[32–35] Yet parents of a suddenly ill child may have no clear idea of what a good parent should do in such circumstances, and no actionable plan of how to go about being that good parent. Spouses, siblings, adult children, and other surrogate decision makers may experience similar confusion about how they can fulfill their defined role in relation to the loved one with a serious illness.[19,24,36] This uncertainty about what they ought to do can bring down an avalanche of negative self-judgment.

Being a parent is often a core part of one's identity once one has children. When a child becomes sick, other goals and identities are often downgraded or dropped.[30,31] Surrogates may experience high levels of anticipated regret as they worry about the consequences of making the wrong decision.[20,37-39] Parents may feel that they have already failed in their obligation to keep their child safe, healthy, and free from harm.[25] This may lead parents to decide, based on their rubric of what would constitute being a "good parent," that a "good parent" never gives up. Even when some parents are painfully aware that a decision may result in suffering for the child, they may be sadly unable to see any other way to fulfill their duty.

In addition to self-judgment, individuals usually have ideas about how others judge them. They may strategically choose to present themselves in a way to avoid expected harsh judgments.[40-43] People anticipate how they think others will perceive them and may change their decisions accordingly.[44] Parents, especially mothers, are used to being judged by others for their decisions and behaviors, even before the child is born.[45]

These social pressures do not go away when a loved one is hospitalized. In the context of serious illness, parents report the importance to them not only of being a good parent but also that others recognize how hard they are working to be a good parent.[30] Surrogates report worrying about what clinicians will think of them if they make the "wrong" decision or argue too much.[20,23,36-38] They also feel a contradictory impulse to advocate for their child and not assume that the staff always know best.[46] Surrogates may not show their full range of thoughts about what they should or should not do, their doubts and fears, or their negative self-judgments. They often wait for the doctors to leave the room and then converse quietly in private. Some keep entirely to themselves. Some only confide in nurses.

Professionals who seek to support fully informed and shared decision making must engage with surrogates' internal monologues about being "good parents," "good sons," "good daughters," and "good spouses." Doing so while avoiding paternalistic judgments of parents is challenging. A medical professional is on safe familiar ground when reviewing the pros and cons of different treatment options. Raising the issue of what "good parents" and "good surrogates" ought to do in a difficult situation may seem judgmental. But everyone grapples with these questions. The clinician cannot ignore them, but mustn't judge. Instead, the goal is to help surrogate decision makers address these questions for themselves and then help them examine their own heuristics and the ways that those can sometimes lead to inappropriately harsh self-judgments.

Epilogue

Later that day, my partner and I left the hospital. We had made our decision and had talked with the medical team. They had outlined when things would happen. Nothing would happen until tomorrow. So after spending a few hours with our daughter, we headed home, trying to prepare ourselves for whatever would happen next.

The medical decision-making process for parents—and more generally, for surrogate decision makers—needs a broader conceptualization, such as we have offered in part here, if we are to adequately meet the needs of surrogate decision makers. While we can suggest sets of questions that can be used to explore aspects of the decision-making process (Table 2.2), much work is needed to determine the most helpful and effective ways to support surrogate decision makers as they engage in the more fully conceptualized process of making medical decisions.

Table 2.2 Questions to Explore Different Aspects of Decision Making

Questions	Aspects of Decision Making Explored
• What do you think are the main problems for [the patient]? • How about for you and your family— what are the main problems?	Problem structuring Situational sensemaking
• What worries you the most? • What are you hoping for?	Problem structuring Preferences, both negative and positive
• Regarding [the patient's] situation, how do you think that we got to where we are now? • Do you think any of the decisions we have made thus far have been mistakes? • Do you have any regrets?	Situational sensemaking Path dependencies Self-judgments
• What do you feel you most need to do to be, in your own judgment, a good [parent, spouse, son, etc.]? • What do you think is most important for you to focus on? • How do you think you are doing?	Personal sense of duty Set of responsibilities Personal operational rules Self-judgments
• How do you think we, the health care team, are getting along with you? • How could we help you better?	Concerns about judgments by others Clarifying collaboration expectations

References

1. Brock DW. Good decisionmaking for incompetent patients. *Hastings Center Rpt*. 1994;24(6):S8–S11.
2. Shalowitz DI, Garrett-Mayer E, Wendler D. The accuracy of surrogate decision makers: a systematic review. *Arch Intern Med*. 2006;166(5):493–497.
3. Charles C, Gafni A, Whelan T. Shared decision-making in the medical encounter: what does it mean? (or it takes at least two to tango). *Social Sci Med (1982)*. 1997;44(5):681–692.
4. Fiks AG, Jimenez ME. The promise of shared decision-making in paediatrics. *Acta Paediatr*. 2010;99(10):1464–1466.
5. van Nistelrooij I, Visse M, Spekkink A, de Lange J. How shared is shared decision-making? A care-ethical view on the role of partner and family. *J Med Ethics*. 2017;43(9):637–644.

6. Whitney SN. A new model of medical decisions: exploring the limits of shared decision making. *Med Decis Mak.* 2003;23(4):275–280.
7. Hill DL, Miller VA, Hexem KR, et al. Problems and hopes perceived by mothers, fathers and physicians of children receiving palliative care. *Health Expect.* 2013.
8. Hill DL, Nathanson PG, Fenderson RM, Carroll KW, Feudtner C. Parental concordance regarding problems and hopes for seriously ill children: a two-year cohort study. *J Pain Symptom Manage.* 2017.
9. Scheunemann LP, Arnold RM, White DB. The facilitated values history: helping surrogates make authentic decisions for incapacitated patients with advanced illness. *Am J Respir Crit Care Med.* 2012;186(6):480–486.
10. Wiener L, Ballard E, Brennan T, Battles H, Martinez P, Pao M. How I wish to be remembered: the use of an advance care planning document in adolescent and young adult populations. *J Palliat Med.* 2008;11(10):1309–1313.
11. Madrigal VN, Carroll KW, Hexem KR, Faerber JA, Morrison WE, Feudtner C. Parental decision-making preferences in the pediatric intensive care unit. *Crit Care Med.* 2012;40(10):2876–2882.
12. Cox CE, Lewis CL, Hanson LC, et al. Development and pilot testing of a decision aid for surrogates of patients with prolonged mechanical ventilation. *Crit Care Med.* 2012;40(8):2327–2334.
13. LeBlanc A, Kenny DA, O'Connor AM, Legare F. Decisional conflict in patients and their physicians: a dyadic approach to shared decision making. *Med Decis Mak.* 2009;29(1):61–68.
14. Nicolai J, Buchholz A, Seefried N, et al. When do cancer patients regret their treatment decision? A path analysis of the influence of clinicians' communication styles and the match of decision-making styles on decision regret. *Patient Educ Couns.* 2016;99(5):739–746.
15. Handy CM, Sulmasy DP, Merkel CK, Ury WA. The surrogate's experience in authorizing a do not resuscitate order. *Palliat Support Care.* 2008;6(1):13–19.
16. Chambers-Evans J, Carnevale FA. Dawning of awareness: the experience of surrogate decision making at the end of life. *J Clinical Ethics.* 2005;16(1):28–45.
17. Radwany S, Albanese T, Clough L, Sims L, Mason H, Jahangiri S. End-of-life decision making and emotional burden: placing family meetings in context. *Am J Hosp Palliat Care.* 2009;26(5):376–383.
18. Wendler D, Rid A. Systematic review: the effect on surrogates of making treatment decisions for others. *Ann Intern Med.* 2011;154(5):336–346.
19. Schenker Y, Crowley-Matoka M, Dohan D, Tiver GA, Arnold RM, White DB. I don't want to be the one saying "we should just let him die": intrapersonal tensions experienced by surrogate decision makers in the ICU. *J Gen Intern Med.* 2012;27(12):1657–1665.

20. Joseph-Williams N, Elwyn G, Edwards A. Knowledge is not power for patients: a systematic review and thematic synthesis of patient-reported barriers and facilitators to shared decision making. *Patient Educ Couns.* 2014;94(3):291–309.

21. Thoits PA. On merging identity theory and stress research. *Soc Psychol Q.* 1991;54(2):101–112.

22. Thoits PA. Role-identity salience, purpose and meaning in life, and well-being among volunteers. *Soc Psychol Q.* 2012;75(4):360–384.

23. Su CT, McMahan RD, Williams BA, Sharma RK, Sudore RL. Family matters: effects of birth order, culture, and family dynamics on surrogate decision-making. *J Am Geriatr Soc.* 2014;62(1):175–182.

24. Majesko A, Hong SH, Weissfeld L, White DB. Identifying family members who may struggle in the role of surrogate decision maker. *Crit Care Med.* 2012;40(8):2281–2286.

25. Horowitz JA. A conceptualization of parenting: examining the single parent family. *Marriage Fam Rev.* 1995;20(1–2):43.

26. Hinds PS, Oakes LL, Hicks J, et al. "Trying to be a good parent" as defined by interviews with parents who made phase I, terminal care, and resuscitation decisions for their children. *J Clin Oncol.* 2009;27(35):5979–5985.

27. October TW, Fisher KR, Feudtner C, Hinds PS. The parent perspective: "being a good parent" when making critical decisions in the PICU. *Pediatr Crit Care Med.* 2014.

28. Feudtner C, Walter JK, Faerber JA, et al. Good-parent beliefs of parents of seriously ill children. *JAMA Pediatr.* 2015;169(1):39–47.

29. Renjilian CB, Womer JW, Carroll KW, Kang TI, Feudtner C. Parental explicit heuristics in decision-making for children with life-threatening illnesses. *Pediatrics.* 2013;131(2):e566–e572.

30. Woodgate RL, Edwards M, Ripat JD, Borton B, Rempel G. Intense parenting: a qualitative study detailing the experiences of parenting children with complex care needs. *BMC Pediatr.* 2015;15:197.

31. Young B, Dixon-Woods M, Findlay M, Heney D. Parenting in a crisis: conceptualising mothers of children with cancer. *Social Sci Med (1982).* 2002;55(10):1835–1847.

32. Higgins ET. Self-discrepancy: a theory relating self and affect. *Psychol Rev.* 1987;94(3):319–340.

33. Markus H, Nurius P. Possible selves. *Am Psychol.* 1986;41(9):954–969.

34. Eisenstadt D, Leippe MR. The self-comparison process and self-discrepant feedback: consequences of learning you are what you thought you were not. *J Pers Social Psychol.* 1994;67(4):611–626.

35. Ogilvie DM. The undesired self: a neglected variable in personality research. *J Pers Social Psychol.* 1987;52(2):379–385.

36. Eves MM, Esplin BS. "She just doesn't know him like we do": illuminating complexities in surrogate decision making. *J Clin Ethics.* 2015;26(4):350–354.

37. Becerra Perez MM, Menear M, Brehaut JC, Legare F. Extent and predictors of decision regret about health care decisions: a systematic review. *Med Decis Making.* 2016;36(6):777–790.

38. de Vos MA, Seeber AA, Gevers SK, Bos AP, Gevers F, Willems DL. Parents who wish no further treatment for their child. *J Med Ethics.* 2015;41(2):195–200.

39. Weiner JS, Roth J. Avoiding iatrogenic harm to patient and family while discussing goals of care near the end of life. *J Palliat Med.* 2006;9(2):451–463.

40. Goffman E. The presentation of self in everyday life. In: Branaman A, ed. *Self and Society.* Malden, MA: Blackwell Publishing; 2001:175–182.

41. Kowalski RM, Leary MR. Strategic self-presentation and the avoidance of aversive events: antecedents and consequences of self-enhancement and self-depreciation. *J Exper Soc Psychol.* 1990;26(4):322–336.

42. Leary MR, Kowalski RM. Impression management: a literature review and two-component model. *Psychol Bull.* 1990;107(1):34–47.

43. Schlenker BR. Self-presentation: managing the impression of consistency when reality interferes with self-enhancement. *J Pers Soc Psychol.* 1975;32(6):1030–1037.

44. Rom SC, Weiss A, Conway P. Judging those who judge: perceivers infer the roles of affect and cognition underpinning others' moral dilemma responses. *J Exper Soc Psychol.* 2017;69:44–58.

45. Burton-Jeangros C. Surveillance of risks in everyday life: the agency of pregnant women and its limitations. *Soc Theor Health.* 2011;9(4):419–436.

46. Kars MC, Duijnstee MS, Pool A, van Delden JJ, Grypdonck MH. Being there: parenting the child with acute lymphoblastic leukaemia. *J Clin Nurs.* 2008;17(12):1553–1562.

3

Clinical Medical Ethics and the Historical Background of Shared Decision Making

Mark Siegler

Shared decision making has become an essential element of the doctor-patient relationship. It was not always so. Over the last 50 years, there has been a vigorous dialogue among doctors, patients, lawyers, philosophers, theologians, and social scientists about the best way for doctors and patients to make decisions together. The complexities are inherent in the asymmetric nature of the doctor-patient relationship. Patients are sick, scared, and vulnerable. Doctors have specialized knowledge and societal privileges and control access to medical resources. Doctors are supposed to serve their patients, but patients often do not and cannot know what they want or need except through the doctors' assistance and guidance. The issues that arise, then, in complex discussions and negotiations between doctors and patients are value laden.

The emergence of the new field of clinical medical ethics (CME) · in the 1970s is closely tied to the development of shared decision making in the early 1980s. In this chapter, I will link the rise of the field of CME with new ideas about shared decision making. I will show how shared decision making reflects a particular view of doctors' moral obligations to both respect patient autonomy and respect their fundamental commitment to use their medical knowledge to improve patients' clinical outcomes.

The Development of the Field of Clinical Medical Ethics

In 1972, I was asked to establish the first intensive care unit at the University of Chicago. There were no "intensivists" at that time. The Society of Critical Care Specialists was only formed in 1970 and critical care medicine would not become a recognized specialty until 1987.

My team and I recognized that doctors who care for critically ill patients needed to think of the ethical aspects of care as an intrinsic part of daily medical practice. We did not think that doing so required the creation of a new academic discipline. We realized that, to do so, we needed to incorporate insights from moral philosophy, law, religion, and anthropology. Still, we saw the ethical considerations in our work primarily as an outgrowth of clinical medicine, as a central component of the clinical care that is practiced and applied by clinicians in their ordinary daily encounters with patients. This was an unusual point of view at the time.

Bioethics itself was a relatively new field, having started in the United States in the mid-1960s. The leading figures in the field were mostly theologians and philosophers. Much of bioethics focused on research ethics questions such as those raised by the Tuskegee syphilis study or those raised by innovative technologies such as in vitro fertilization. By contrast, my team called attention to the ways in which ethical issues arose in the everyday practice of medicine. Eventually, we described what we were doing as CME.

During the past 47 years, I have been delighted to see that CME has gradually become integrated into medical education and medical practice. Done right, it can improve the clinical and ethical quality of both routine and complex care. CME does this by addressing issues like truth telling, informed consent, confidentiality, surrogate decision making, and end-of-life choices. CME encourages personal, humane, compassionate, and fair interactions between doctor and patient. The editors of the *Lancet* recognized the power and the importance of CME in a powerful editorial in 1997: "Debate on ethical matters is as much an integral part of everyday doctoring as choosing the best treatment for patients."[1]

We faced a challenge in engaging clinicians in these discussions and reflections. There was widespread ignorance among clinicians about the new field of bioethics. Many clinicians were skeptical about the value of philosophy or theology for dilemmas that arose in the clinical setting. Some were overtly hostile and saw philosophers as meddlers or as external critics of the practice of medicine. To bridge this unfortunate gap between thoughtful people who were all trying to do their best for patients, I chose to dedicate my career to teaching clinicians how to integrate ethical reasoning into their everyday clinical practices.

In 1974, James Gustafson, legal scholar Ann Dudley Goldblatt, and I were funded by the Department of Health, Education, and Welfare to develop a multidisciplinary program in CME at the University of Chicago. This was the first grant application, federal or otherwise, to use the term "clinical ethics."

Several years later, I suggested that the bedside teaching of clinical ethics was not at all new. In fact, I showed, it was a legacy of William Osler.[2] This article was well received and, in 1979, I was invited to start a section on CME in the AMA's *Archives of Internal Medicine*.[3]

These efforts introduced clinical ethics to physicians. Many began to recognize the importance of the new discipline for their work with patients. They began to understand that informed consent was complicated, that truth telling was not always straightforward, and that end-of-life decisions often raised profound spiritual, emotional, legal, and philosophical questions. The field of CME brought insights from all these fields together.

This new prominence for CME generated a backlash. In 1996, Daniel Callahan, cofounder of the Hastings Center and one of the early leaders in the American bioethics movement, strongly criticized CME. Callahan stated: "In one of my first articles on bioethics, I wrote that the principal aim of the field should be to help the medical practitioner deal with concrete cases. While I would hardly want to overlook the needs of the practitioner, I now wonder if that is the right place to center our attention.... Does reality lie in the particularity of individual cases where most clinicians think it does—or in a more general, abstract and universal realm, no less real but just more hidden?"[4]

The year after Callahan's article was published in *The Hastings Center Report*, the *Lancet* published an editorial that strongly disagreed with Callahan's views. They stated: "Ethics needs to be rooted in clinical practice and not in armchair moral philosophy. Debate on ethical matters is as much an integral part of everyday doctoring as choosing the best treatment for patients. Departments of ethics that are divorced from the medical profession, wallowing in theory and speculation, are all quaintly redundant."[1]

Following Callahan's critique and the *Lancet* editorial, the New York Academy of Medicine convened a conference, in 1980, to examine some of the issues raised by the debate between philosophers like Callahan and physicians like myself and those who wrote for the *Lancet*.

A Meeting of the New York Academy of Medicine

The 1980 Annual Conference of the New York Academy of Medicine focused on the topic "The Patient and the Healthcare Professional: The Changing Pattern of Their Relationship."[5] They noted that physician paternalism, rooted in the principle of benefi-cence, had been the dominant model of doctor-patient encounters for thousands of years. But paternalism was on the wane, crumbling beneath a philosophical critique that emphasized the over-whelming importance of patient autonomy. The tension between paternalism and autonomy reverberated in discussions ranging from informed consent to decision making for dying patients to ethically desirable models of the physician-patient relationship. Autonomy and paternalism were often in conflict. In medicine, traditional paternalism assumed great moral authority because good health was assumed to be a value shared by the patient and the physician and because physicians' knowledge and clinical abilities placed them in a position to help patients regain good health. The paternalism model emphasized patient care rather than patient wishes, patient needs rather than their rights, and physician competence rather than patient autonomy. The new focus on autonomy was driven by political and social movements that aimed to gain entitlements and rights, to achieve equity and equality in the distribution of health services, and to reduce the hierarchical barrier between patient and physician.

At that conference, I argued that the central moral and practical dilemma facing patients and physicians was to balance the rights of patients and the responsibilities of physicians—and the rights of physicians and the responsibilities of patients—at a time when societal values were changing. To do so, I suggested, we needed to find some middle ground. That middle ground, I suggested, was most likely to be discovered in the particularities of the interactions between physicians and patients as they worked together to make decisions about diagnostic testing and treatment. I called those interactions "the doctor-patient accommodation." Today, they might be called "shared decision making."

The goal of both the doctor-patient accommodation and shared decision making is to develop a bilateral model in which the moral and technical arrangements of a medical encounter are determined mutually, voluntarily, and autonomously by both patient and physician. This bilateral accommodation model would overcome the unilateral, static notion of either a physician-dominated paternalistic model or a patient-dominated autonomy-libertarian model of medicine.[7]

The physician-patient accommodation is both a process and an outcome. Beginning with the initial encounter between patient and physician, there is a degree of testing by both parties to decide whether this patient and this physician can work together to benefit the patient. The process is one of communication, negotiation, and joint decision making as to what rights and responsibilities each of the parties wishes to retain and which would be relinquished in the context of their medical relationship. When it works, ". . . a joint decision is reached on whether this patient and this physician will work together to address the patient's health concerns."[6]

Two years after the conference at the New York Academy of Medicine, the President's Commission for the Study of Ethical Problems in Medicine endorsed the concept of the patient-physician accommodation and linked it to the idea of shared decision making. They recommended fostering a patient-physician relationship "characterized by mutual participation and respect and by *shared decision making*. The Commission believes such a shift in focus will do better justice to the realities of health care and to the ethical values underlying the informed consent doctrine."[7]

Following the commission's report in 1982, shared decision making has become the prevailing model of decision making in the US health care system. The key element of shared decision making is that it is neither pure paternalism nor unadulterated autonomy. By the early 2000s, empirical evidence began to accumulate showing that most doctors and patients prefer the middle ground. Murray and colleagues illustrated this in a national survey of doctors and patients that showed that 62% of patients and 75% of doctors preferred shared decision making over autonomy-consumerism or paternalism.[8,9]

Shared Decision Making and Clinical Medical Ethics

The rise of shared decision making reflects some insights that were originally addressed by the field of CME. Those insights draw on four essential features of CME.

First, CME is a discipline of medicine, not of legal, theological, or philosophical bioethics. Good patient care requires that treatment and scientific considerations be integrated with personal and ethical considerations. Ethical concerns have always been an essential part of medical practice—from Hippocrates to John Gregory to Thomas Percival to Richard Cabot to Francis Peabody to the present. The extraordinary scientific achievements of the past 75 years have increased the range, intensity, and frequency of ethical issues in medicine and have encouraged the development of CME as an integral component of daily medical practice. And an essential component of CME is doctor-patient communication around ethically complex situations and choices.

A second essential element of CME relates to medical education. The formation of professional identity as a physician requires attention to the inherently ethical aspects of clinical medicine. The main goal in teaching CME to medical students and residents is not to help them understand moral theory, but rather to improve the quality of patient care in terms of both the process and outcome of care by integrating ethical issues into clinical reasoning. We teach CME to medical students because they must, every day, in every clinical encounter, engage in a complex process of shared decision making with their patients. When this is done right, it leads to high-quality medicine, greater patient satisfaction, and better clinical outcomes.

Third, the foundation of CME is the doctor-patient encounter. This encounter is at the heart of medicine and always has been. Sick people seek healers because the relationship between a healer and a sufferer meets universal and unchanging human needs. For complex reasons, the nature of that encounter has changed, even though the essential need for it has not. Both the paternalism and autonomy models imply an adversarial relationship between the physician and patient, although the models disagree on whether the ultimate power and control should rest in the doctor's hands or the patient's hands. By contrast, the field of CME aims to improve patient outcomes by supporting and defending a patient-centered focus in medical practice that encourages a process of nonadversarial, shared decision making between patients and physicians.

Finally, CME is an empirical discipline. Research is essential to test hypotheses and improve outcomes. The research work of CME differs greatly from the philosophical-analytic research of traditional bioethics. CME research often employs the methods of clinical epidemiology, decision analysis, evidence-based outcomes, and health services research to gather empirical data to reach conclusions about such ethical issues as end-of-life care, the patient's quality of life, parental choices in newborn intensive care units, organ transplantation, and the core elements of the doctor-patient relationship. Empirical data showing that a particular way of ethical practice is better than the alternative helps develop a professional consensus and leads to changes in medical practice. Previously, ethics research had relied upon non-data-based analytical scholarship done by theologians, legal scholars, and bioethicists, and such analytic scholarship had less success in modifying clinical practice than empirical data-driven clinical studies. In 1996, Wennberg summarized the role of empirical research for the study of decision making: "It is the job of the evaluative sciences to conduct technology assessment and outcomes research to estimate the probability for outcomes that matter to patients and to elucidate the importance of patient preferences in choosing treatment."[10]

Over the years, empirical studies have confirmed that a process of shared decision making improves patient care in each of the following ways:

- Patients have greater trust and confidence in their doctors.
- Patients comply better with treatment plans that they have agreed upon with their doctors.
- Patients have greater satisfaction with their care.
- Doctors and patients reach more appropriate financial decisions.
- In a number of chronic diseases, including hypertension, diabetes, arthritis, and depression, patients experience better outcomes.

These outcomes and goals are the goals of CME. They set clinical-ethical standards that have become the legal and professional standard of care in the United States. CME integrates ethical principles with routine daily clinical practice. CME requires the commitment and involvement of both patients and clinicians, who work together through the process of shared decision making to improve medical practice and patient outcomes. As we look toward the future and recognize emerging challenges to humane, compassionate, and personalized medical practice, we will need to continually emphasize the central importance of the doctor-patient relationship and vigorously support the model of shared decision making between patients and doctors.

References

1. Lancet Editorial Board. The ethics industry. *Lancet.* 1997;350(9082):897.
2. Siegler M. A legacy of Osler: teaching clinical ethics at the bedside. *JAMA.* 1978;239:951–956.
3. Siegler M. Clinical ethics and clinical medicine. *Arch Int Med.* 1979;139:914–915.

4. Callahan D. Does clinical ethics distort the discipline? *Hast Ctr Rep.* 1996;26 (6):28–29.
5. The patient and the health care professional: the changing pattern of their relations. *Bull NY Acad Med.* 1981;57:1–86.
6. Siegler M. Searching for moral certainty in medicine. *Bull N Y Acad Med.* 1981;57(1):56–69.
7. President's Commission for the Study of Ethical Problems in Medicine and Biomedical and Behavioral Research. Making health care decisions: a report on the ethical and legal implications of informed consent in the patient-practitioner relationship, volume one: report. October 1982:36–37.   https://repository.library.georgetown.edu/bitstream/handle/10822/559354/making_health_care_decisions.pdf?sequence=1&isAllowed=y. Accessed April 25, 2019.
8. Murray E, Pollack L, White M, Lo B. Clinical decision-making: patients' preferences and experiences. *Patient Educ Counsel.* 2007;65:189–196.
9. Murray E, Pollack L, White M, Lo B. Clinical decision-making: physicians' preferences and experiences. *BMC Fam Pract.* 2007;8:1–10.
10. Wennberg J. Social and economic issues in medicine. In: Plum F, Bennet JC, eds. *Cecil Textbook of Medicine.* 20th ed. Philadelphia: TOREW.B.Saunders Co; 1996:54.

4

Practical Wisdom, Rules, and the Patient-Doctor Conversation

Daniel Brudney

Well, it is thought characteristic of a wise person to be able to deliberate well about the things that are good and advantageous to himself, not in specific contexts, e.g., what sorts of things conduce to health or to physical strength, but what sorts of things conduce to the good life in general.
—Aristotle, *Nicomachean Ethics* 1140a25–29

In this chapter, I explore what I take to be a tension between one of the aspirations of the standard algorithm for decision making at the bedside and what often actually happens there.[1] The aspiration in question is to avoid physician paternalism, but the algorithm seems also to try to exclude the physician's exercise of their capacity for a crucial element of what philosophers call "practical reason." Now, the exercise of any capacity includes the possibility of exercising it well. With practical reason, this means getting things right. It amounts to having "practical wisdom" about the issue at hand. The current algorithm for bedside decision making has had the effect of limiting the scope for the exercise of the physician's practical wisdom—and yet such exercise is what clinical practice sometimes requires.

The Flight From Practical Wisdom

There are many reasons for the shift from the physician paternalist to the patient autonomy model. The most obvious is the belief that individuals have a moral right to run their own lives—the patient's right to decide is merely an instance of this broader moral right. But there is another reason, namely, skepticism that physicians are wiser than others in their normative judgments at the bedside. The phrase from back in the day, "Doctor knows best," was not a claim solely about technical knowledge. It also expressed the belief that the physician's overall bedside judgment—including both technical and normative content—was better than that of anyone else on the scene. The physician was thought to be "wise."

A quick argument for medical paternalism goes as follows:

> Premise 1: One's goal is the best overall outcome for the patient.
> Premise 2: Determining what is likely to be the best overall outcome for the patient requires the exercise of practical wisdom; that is, it requires the excellent exercise of practical reason.
> Premise 3: The exercise of practical wisdom requires a person who possesses practical wisdom.
> Premise 4: Among those at the bedside, with regard to the decision at hand, the person most likely to be a person of practical wisdom is the physician.
> Conclusion: The physician should make the bedside decision.

I think the demise of paternalism was due in part to increasing skepticism about Premise 4.[2] Call this "doctor-knows-best skepticism."

To see where such skepticism fits into clinical practice, let's examine the current algorithm for bedside decision making. At step

1, there is a patient-doctor conversation, and then the patient decides to accept or to refuse this or that recommended treatment option. The criterion for whether to accept the patient's decision is not whether their decision is wise or foolish but whether they have decisional capacity. We hope that the patient has good judgment, although we know this is often not the case.

If the patient does not have decisional capacity, a surrogate decides. The first thing the surrogate is supposed to do (step 2) is to determine whether the patient has ever indicated their decision with regard to the treatment at issue, through an advance directive or in some other way. At step 2, the surrogate is functioning as a witness. They are not being asked to make a normative judgment but only a factual judgment. They are not required to possess practical wisdom.

If the patient did not indicate their decision about the treatment at issue, we get to step 3. Here, the surrogate is supposed to answer a different question, the "What would the patient choose in this situation?" question. Here too at stake is something factual, namely, the surrogate's knowledge of the patient's beliefs and values. The surrogate is not asked to judge whether they are wise or foolish. They are asked only to use their knowledge of the patient to determine what the patient would have decided. Again, practical wisdom is not required.

It is only if there is no answer to the "What would the patient choose?" question that we get to step 4, and the surrogate is asked to determine which option is in the patient's best interests. This does seem to require good judgment, that is, practical wisdom. Even here, however, the scope for such judgment is restricted. The surrogate is supposed to judge only which option is best for the patient. Other considerations are not supposed to intrude.[3] Moreover, and crucially, there seems to be no role for the exercise of the physician's practical wisdom.

General Rules and Particular Judgments

Skepticism about the physician's special possession of practical wisdom seems to restrict the physician from engaging in any serious moral deliberation about what is best for the patient. One source of this restriction on physician practical wisdom might be what Paul Ricoeur calls "the hermeneutics of suspicion"—the thought that any claim to be wise is a cover for class prejudice or race prejudice or some other form of individual or group interest.[4] Moreover, there might be skepticism about the practical wisdom specifically of institutionally assigned decision makers such as doctors. They might be thought to be subject to a range of pressures likely either to distort their judgment or to undermine their willingness to exercise it properly.

Putting such speculation aside, what needs to be stressed is that a lack of confidence in the wisdom of a particular group of decision makers does not entail a lack of confidence in every decision maker of the relevant kind. The lack of confidence is usually in the average decision maker. Consider a rule that prohibits any surgeon from operating the morning after a night in which they have been on call. Assume the justification for the rule is compelling data that shows that, after having been up all night, the average surgeon is not able to judge their own surgical competence. (For our purposes, it is not relevant whether the data actually shows this.) Given the stipulated data, and given that avoiding bad surgical outcomes is more important than the inconvenience to patients of rescheduling surgery, it might make sense to impose this rule. Yet there need be no assumption that every surgeon is unable to make a good judgment. When Dr. Smith says that she does not need such a rule because she knows when she is unfit to operate, she might be correct, but the rule was not made with her in mind. It was made for the many surgeons who are not to be relied on to judge correctly when they are unfit to operate. The inconvenience the rule imposes on Dr. Smith and her patients is collateral damage. There is simply no viable mechanism to protect the patients of surgeons who are not as self-aware as Dr. Smith without inconveniencing the patients of surgeons who are.

Philosophers call this "rule consequentialism." That doctrine holds that one should do the action such that, if the action were made into a rule with widespread compliance, better consequences would result than would result from compliance with any other relevant and feasible rule.[5]

Philosophers have long known that the rule that yields the best overall consequences might yield suboptimal consequences in individual cases. Consider the rule that mandates rigid confidentiality about the results of HIV tests. At the beginning of the AIDS epidemic, public health officials believed that the most important thing to do was to get people tested, and that only the promise of confidentiality would induce people to come in for testing. That the confidentiality rule was the right rule at the time is consistent with conceding that in some cases it might have had problematic consequences. In some cases, a doctor might have known that a patient was HIV positive but was not permitted to inform the patient's sexual partner, who might have been in the waiting room. This might have led to avoidable infection and, in those days, even avoidable death. Endorsing the propriety of the rigid confidentiality rule is consistent with conceding that it did not produce the best outcome in every case.

It often makes sense to use a rule even if it doesn't produce the best outcome in every case. This can create a puzzle. In thinking about doctor-knows-best skepticism, it can seem a good rule to assume that, in the clinical setting, the doctor is not the wisest person at the bedside and that, therefore, they ought to defer to the judgment of the patient, surrogate, or parent. Yet one could simultaneously accept that, at times, the doctor might be the wisest person there and would make the best decision. The puzzle is that it might sometimes be right to violate the rule, but there is no reliable way to know when.

The Physician-Patient Conversation

Despite the standard decision algorithm, doctors do often try to bring practical wisdom to bear. How could they not? The patient, surrogate, or parent needs help, and merely offering information is not sufficient. The need is for advice, for counsel, but to give advice or counsel is to claim at least a little practical wisdom. In clinical life the need for the physician to have practical wisdom works its way back in, and it is in the hardest cases that the need is greatest. So we get to shared decision making.

Now, there are many models of shared decision making.[6] Rather than try to adjudicate among them, I would like, instead, to examine some elements of the patient-doctor conversation and then adapt these elements to the pediatric setting. Shared decision making involves a conversation that can be seen as a joint exercise of practical reason. Physician and patient (or surrogate) reason together. In trying to determine how such reasoning might be done well, we can ask which of the (many) traditional elements of practical reason ought to be involved. I list three.

- Element 1 is reasoning about the various parts of a given end or goal and how they fit together as well as reasoning about how one's various goals fit together. It is rational to understand what one is after and to determine how far pursuing goal A will facilitate or undermine pursuing goals B or C.
- Element 2 is reasoning about the proper goal or goals to have, either in a given situation or for a life as a whole. This sometimes goes under the heading of reasoning or deliberating about the content of the good for a human being or, more commonly, the good for a particular person. This is not an arcane enterprise. One does it all the time. For example, in raising children, one might make choices about schools as well as about soccer versus baseball versus violin versus

ballet, etc. In these decisions one is judging what is likely to be good for one's child.
- Element 3 arises once one has settled on a goal. One then engages in reasoning about how to attain it. This is "instrumental reasoning" or "means-and-ends reasoning."

Thinking first about the adult patient, here it seems clear that clinicians are engaged in practical reasoning in the sense of means-and-ends reasoning. They are trained to know which treatments have which probability of leading to which outcome. As for element 1, goal specification, this is primarily the province of the patient. At stake are the goals of care as well as the clarification of values that might be involved in deciding upon those goals. Here, the clinician's role is to facilitate the patient's understanding of their values and goals so that they can be in a position to evaluate their medical options.

What about element 2, reasoning about the human good, specifically reasoning about the good for this patient in front of the clinician? I take doctor-knows-best skepticism to be skepticism that the doctor is better than the patient at element 2. A decision-making algorithm that tries to minimize or even to eliminate the doctor as engaged in deliberating with the patient about the good is based on the premise that, on average, clinicians are not wiser about such things than the patient. The force of this—by now old—point is that it is best to have the rule that patient choice, not physician choice, is the basis of treatment.

Yet even if the doctor is usually not wiser than the patient, sometimes they might be. (See the discussion in General Rules and Particular Judgments.) Imagine a newly disabled patient who satisfies the criteria for decisional capacity and yet feels that life with her disability is not worth living and so refuses life-sustaining treatment. Her doctor might believe that, with more time, she would come to find new activities valuable and satisfying. Her values would change. She would come to see that her life could be well worth living. To take another example, Julian Savelescu has written about a patient with breast cancer who refused the surgery that, at that time, held the best chance for her to live because she worried it would make her unattractive to her husband. Savelescu claimed that it was proper for her doctor to challenge the values leading to this decision.[7] Savelescu's claim was that element 2 (beliefs about values, about the human good) could be a proper topic for the patient-doctor conversation.

Consider the following thoughts:

(1) Doctors are usually less wise about the proper goals of a patient's life than the patient;
(2) The doctor is sometimes wiser about these goals than the patient; and
(3) The doctor is wise enough to know when they are wiser about these goals.

Most people would probably accept (1) and (2). Now, (1) and (3) are not logically incompatible, but someone who subscribes to (1) might be skeptical about (3). Yet only if (3) is true, only if the doctor knows when they are likely to be wiser than the patient, is the doctor ever justified in pushing back against what they think are worrisome patient values. And one might think that the doctor is sometimes justified.

The Parent-Pediatrician Conversation

Let's shift now to the conversation between parent and pediatrician. This too is a joint exercise of practical reason. Here too the issue of physician practical wisdom can arise. Consider two possible goals of the parent-pediatrician conversation.

Goal A: The goal is to inform the parent of the options for the child patient and to help the parent clarify their thinking. It is assumed that the parent knows best what the proper ends for their child are.

Goal B: The goal is jointly to determine the overall best thing to do for the child patient. The parent is the final decision maker, but both parties have serious input into determining the proper ends for the child (element 2 earlier). Together, they are trying to decide in the way that a person with practical wisdom would decide.

Note that Goal B does not completely reject Goal A. Rather, to the tasks of presenting options and helping to clarify thinking, it adds the task of jointly finding the overall best thing to do. Element 2 is part of the conversation.[8]

One difference between the adult and the pediatric setting is that, in the latter, element 2 is, to some extent, legally embedded in the conversation. The pediatrician has a duty to make sure that the child's interests are not excessively compromised, for instance, that the child is not the victim of medical abuse or neglect. The parent has leeway to exercise a preference that does not track the child's "best" interests but merely "good enough" interests. Still, there are limits, and it is the pediatrician's duty to monitor them. Deliberation about what is good for the child is always an implicit part of the parent-pediatrician conversation.[9] I suspect that most pediatricians see Goal B as the proper goal of the parent-pediatrician conversation. The pediatrician's patient is the child, not the parent. Helping the parent to make a decision is part of looking after the child's well-being, but the child's well-being, not the exercise of parental autonomy, is the pediatrician's focus.

If the child's well-being is the pediatrician's focus, and if some view of the child's good is necessarily part of looking after the child's well-being, then there will sometimes be a question as to whether the pediatrician should challenge the parent's values. I am imagining a challenge that would go beyond monitoring abuse or neglect and into the sphere in which, legally, the parent has leeway to make the decision.

This question arises if we accept my claims about general rules and particular judgments. Suppose we assume (i) the parent is usually wiser about their child's well-being than the pediatrician, but also (ii) the pediatrician is sometimes wiser. Jointly, (i) and (ii) raise the question of whether the pediatrician is ever entitled—indeed, ever has the duty—to assert that, here and now, with this child patient, the pediatrician is wiser than the parent and so is entitled to push back against the parent's judgment. Most pediatricians likely see themselves as permitted and even obligated sometimes to push back against a parent's judgment. As noted, their primary duty is to the child, not the parent.

It is important to keep two things in mind. First, to endorse this role for the pediatrician is not to return to physician paternalism. Aside from situations of abuse or neglect, the final decision is the parent's. Moreover, the hope is that the parent-pediatrician conversation will involve a good-faith attempt to determine together what would be the best outcome for the child. In practice, such a conversation might be difficult to achieve (it must somehow be insulated from the pediatrician-parent power asymmetry); even so, it is the proper model to try to instantiate.

Nevertheless, second, there does remain a residue of paternalism because, on the account that I have sketched, the pediatrician is sometimes implicitly asserting that they do possess not merely technical knowledge and experience but also practical wisdom about this child patient's good. Such an assertion rejects the premise underlying the standard decision-making algorithm, namely, that doctor doesn't know best. Acting on the implicit assertion that at times, say, here, with this child, doctor does know best is, I think, a crucial part of the pediatrician's job. Yet if we assume that, on average, the parent knows best, then the pediatrician is taking a fraught step in asserting that here and now they know best. The pediatrician might well be wrong. Still, taking that step is sometimes what they are supposed to do. This suggests that there can be a kind of moral challenge (more dramatically, the need for a kind of moral courage) in the pediatrician's job.

I don't think I have said anything that a practicing pediatrician doesn't already know. I have tried simply to excavate the assumptions that lie behind the standard decision-making algorithm and to show how these assumptions can be in tension with a proper understanding of the patient-physician and, here, more specifically, the parent-pediatrician conversation.

References

1. Thanks to Chris Feudtner for suggesting the term "algorithm" here.
2. For a powerful version of this claim, see Veatch RM. Generalization of expertise. *Hastings Ctr Stud.* 1973;1(2):29–40.
3. For the view that the steps presented are a common norm, see *Deciding to Forego Life-Sustaining Treatment: A Report on the Ethical, Medical and Legal Issues in Treatment Decisions,* President's Commission for the Study of Ethical Problems in Medicine and Biomedical and Behavioral Research, March 1983. See chapter II, especially pp. 126–140. See also Brock D, Buchanan A. *Deciding for Others.* Cambridge: Cambridge University Press; 1998: Chapter 2.
4. See Ricoeur R. *Freud and Philosophy: An Essay on Interpretation* (Denis Savage, transl.). New Haven, CT: Yale University Press; 2008:32.
5. For a discussion of rule consequentialism, see the online *Stanford Encyclopedia of Philosophy* entry, https://plato.stanford.edu/entries/consequentialism-rule/.
6. See, for instance, Thomasma DC. Beyond medical paternalism and patient autonomy: a model of physician conscience for the physician-patient relationship. *Ann Intern Med.* 1983;98:243–248. Quill TE. Partnerships in patient care: a contractual approach. *Ann Intern Med.* 1983;98:228–234. Emanuel EJ, Emanuel LL. Four models of the physician-patient relationship. *JAMA.* 1992;267(16):2221–2226. Veatch RM. Models for ethical medicine in a revolutionary age. *Hastings Ctr Rep.* 1972;2(3):5–7.
7. See Savelescu J. Rational non-interventional paternalism: why doctors ought to make judgments of what is best for their patients. *J Med Eth.* 1995;21(6):327–331.
8. An example of the uncertainty about goals in the pediatric setting is Alexander Kon's list of forms of shared decision-making. Kon's analysis puts the weight on noting which party is more responsible for the final

decision rather than on the goal of the conversation. Still, Kon lists five ways in which parents and doctors can combine to reach a decision. Some of these fall on the side of facilitating parental preference, others on the side of searching together for the best outcome. See Kon A. Commentary. *JAMA.* 2010;304(8):903–904.

9. On this topic, see Diekema D. Parental refusals of medical treatment: the harm principle as threshold for state intervention. *Theor Med Bioeth.* 2004;25(4):243–264.

5

Scaffolding Autonomy

Respecting Persons in Shared Decision Making

Jodi Halpern and Aleksa Owen

The goal of shared decision making (SDM) is to honor a patient's autonomy while at the same time recognizing that patients are vulnerable in many ways and may need help to both realize and exercise their right to make decisions for themselves. This is most obvious in cases involving adolescents or adults with mild to moderate intellectual/developmental disabilities (IDDs). But it is present in most medical decisions because of the nature of those decisions. Doctors have expertise that patients need. Patients seek knowledge but also seek guidance in applying that knowledge to their own situations. Clinicians must interpret patients' stated wishes in light of what they know about the patients' clinical situation as well as what they know about each patient's psychosocial situation. Often, multiple clinicians and many family members are involved. It can be hard to know whose autonomy should be prioritized. We must weigh the multiple and often clashing perspectives of clinicians, parents or caregivers, and the patients themselves. The patient's autonomy can get lost in the complex mix of competing interests and perspectives.

To illustrate the ways that a patient's autonomy can get subsumed by the values and preferences of others, we will analyze two cases in which doctors' and parents' beliefs, values, and choices may have undermined their desire to show respect for the patient's autonomy. We explore how this undermining may take place because of physicians' unexamined biases or psychological reactions to the patient's situation. We suggest that, as a field, bioethics sometimes focuses on a narrow interpretation of autonomy that, paradoxically, may distract us from an attempt to understand what is really going on when doctors and patients in an emotionally fraught clinical encounter choose an easier but shallower view of what autonomy means and, by doing so, fail to truly and deeply respect their patients' most deeply held beliefs. We argue that a deep respect for persons should take precedence over respect for the shallow sort of autonomy that is sometimes valued in clinical settings today. This is especially true when circumstances are such that the patients' exercise of their own autonomy is constrained by age, disability, or illness. Respect for persons is the central frame through which empathic communication about medical decision making should occur.

The ongoing debate around the call for SDM revolves around who should actually be making difficult medical decisions. This challenge invokes questions for the clinicians around responsibility, power, and authorization.[1] Rather than focusing on traditional bioethics concerns of a balancing act between too little and too much professional interference, our chapter uses two examples of more complex, multiparty situations to explore how psychological respect for persons, or dignity, can be a facilitator for SDM in contexts where developmental issues may preclude a clear clinical understanding of the person's autonomy.

Adolescents and adults with IDDs are distinct populations with different cognitive frames and abilities and differing levels of autonomy. While one of our cases involves a teen and the other an adult with an IDD, we do not mean to suggest that they are the same or somehow collapse the ethical concerns that arise from working with these two groups. Rather, we want to foreground the space between "full" autonomy (a competent adult) and a complete lack of autonomy (a newborn baby or person with very severe IDD). This in-between space is the ethical space where issues are most complex and where clinicians may struggle the most.

For both adolescents and adults with IDDs, it may not be possible to honor autonomy in the same way that it would be for adults who are considered to have full autonomy. For these patients, there is still a need to prevent either abandoning patients to face difficult decisions alone or having doctors paternalistically take over such decisions. In these cases, the affected individuals and their families need help hearing, processing, and facing difficult, even traumatic, diagnoses and prognoses and coping with poor treatment options. This is not news. Experienced physicians, nurses, and social workers know patients and families need help hearing bad news and facing tragic choices. What we focus on here is how physicians can provide the kind of safety, respect, and support necessary to enable patients and families to think through what is otherwise cognitively overwhelming and emotionally intolerable. In discussing this, our intention is not to address specific communication skills; there is already much written about skillful empathic communication.[2] Rather, we stress three underlying communication conditions necessary to facilitate true SDM.

First, physicians must communicate effectively in light of the distinct cognitive, emotional, and social world of the patient. This requires being well informed about patients' developmental capacities. For example, how an adolescent hears information about life, death, pain, and suffering differs categorically rather than merely quantitatively from how either an adult or a younger child processes such information. In the case of adults with IDDs, their processing might be difficult to understand, prompting a physician to seek insight about the interior world of such a patient from caregivers or family and, whenever possible, from the patients themselves.

Second, physicians must become skillful in recognizing how much their own unconscious emotional projections frame the decisions they offer their patients in the first place. We expand on this concept throughout the chapter.

Third, bioethics needs to better delineate the obligation to respect children, adolescents, and individuals with IDDs as persons even if they are not yet, or will ever be, fully capable of autonomy. For instance, many adults with IDDs may have legal guardians throughout their life, but that should not preclude gaining their assent and full participation in health care decision making. The question, of course, is *how* to practice respect for persons when autonomy is not fully developed. We argue here that the obligation of respecting persons needs to be distinguished from and weighed appropriately against the responsibility to protect the best interests of young adolescents or adults with IDDs, which arises from beneficence.

Case #1: Communicating a Dire Prognosis to a 13-Year-Old

The following tragic case appeared in *Pediatrics* in 2001 with commentary by two pediatricians and an ethicist about what the doctors should do when an adolescent refuses treatment for a life-threatening illness.[3] We recognize that the case describes treatments that are now outdated. Jorge's treatment would be very different today. But our goal in this chapter is not to focus on the clinical aspects of the case but, instead, on the types of discussions that took place. We believe that similar discussions take place today, but in somewhat different clinical contexts.

Jorge, a 13-year-old Hispanic male, was admitted and treated for acute lymphocytic leukemia 9 months ago. He promptly experienced remission in the first month of therapy. This was followed by 6 months of intensive consolidation that required numerous hospitalizations. He then was placed on maintenance chemotherapy.

Jorge is the oldest son of five children born to working-class parents who were both high school graduates.

While undergoing induction, Jorge and his parents seemed to be aware of his treatment course and prognosis. The family related well to the treatment team, and Jorge developed a close relationship with the oncology social worker. At first, he appeared depressed. At times he would state that he was "cursed" and would never live to graduate college, a long-term goal he shared with his family. However, despite his age, Jorge appeared to be quite mature and was always cooperative with medical procedures.

During his second month in maintenance therapy, Jorge was doing well both clinically and socially. His hair was growing back well. He had returned to school for partial-day attendance. His mood was pleasant, and he seemed to be adjusting to resuming life. During a routine clinic visit, a bone marrow aspiration detected the resurgence of his acute lymphocytic leukemia. He and his family were told about this by the oncologist who worked closely with them.

Jorge, his parents, and his two siblings appeared devastated by this news. The oncologist explained that Jorge's only chance for survival would be to receive a bone marrow transplant (BMT). Jorge immediately asked what his chances of living were. He was told that approximately 40% of children would survive and be disease-free for 5 years. After a prolonged consultation during which various options were discussed, his family agreed to visit the transplantation center to get additional information. At the center, they were informed about the lengthy time he would need to be in seclusion, the amount of pain and invasiveness involved with the procedure, the long-term issues about graft-versus-host disease, and the likelihood of success using a partially matched nonrelated donor. His parents reported that Jorge asked very few questions and did not get along well with the supervising oncologist at the transplant referral center.

On returning home, Jorge announced to his parents that he did not want the BMT. His parents, who were absolutely firm that every possible treatment should be pursued, called the oncologist for help. A meeting was arranged the next day, and Jorge and his parents, doctor, social worker, and primary nurse met to discuss the options. His doctor noted that Jorge appeared to be very firm in his decision that he would refuse to cooperate. Jorge had read about other teenagers who had also chosen to die rather than accept additional painful treatments. They felt that a 40% chance was better than no chance at all. They asked his doctor to place Jorge on the waiting list, despite Jorge's strenuous objections. The doctors were not sure what to do.[4]

This is where the case ends and the commentaries by two pediatric oncologists and one bioethicist begin. All three focus solely on what to do next. This focus is typical of bioethical interventions in cases like this where there appears to be an intractable disagreement and a breakdown or impasse in communication. Bioethicists reflect on what to do after a breakdown in communication rather than asking how the breakdown happened in the first place. The commentators make a few suggestions of how to try to change Jorge's mind and then quickly move on to assert the need to respect Jorge's autonomy by accepting his refusal of the transplant.

But the process by which the breakdown occurred might be more helpful both in this case and in cases like this. Certain styles of communication, reflecting certain beliefs about the appropriate way to engage in the process of SDM, may be more likely than others to lead to such disagreements.

Consider the way that each physician communicated with Jorge. First, the oncologist immediately answered Jorge's question about his prognosis with a statistic: 40% survival at 5 years. By beginning with the most emotionally difficult fact, the oncologist almost ensured that Jorge would not be able to process any further information. We suggest that, in such situations, a better process of SDM would have been to first elicit Jorge's understanding of his disease and of the meaning of remission, and then, perhaps, to inquire about Jorge's hopes and fears. Only then, perhaps, would it be time to give—and frame—information in a way that Jorge would be able to make use of.

This physician was doing what the American bioethics movement was calling for at the time, respecting patient autonomy by fully disclosing all requested information. Doctors were being coached not to avoid talking about death with dying children. Not telling them the truth, by this view, could rob them of the opportunity to have meaningful conversations with their parents and the medical team.

Second, soon after Jorge heard this news, he and his family mustered up the hope to go and meet with the transplant team. The transplant doctor emphasized all the negative facts: Jorge would face prolonged seclusion and pain, the risk of graft-versus-host disease, and lower odds of success with an unrelated donor. Although both doctors were dutifully fulfilling their understanding of what respecting Jorge required, such vivid and frightening information clearly terrified the 13-year-old boy.

The SDM paradigm attempts to enable effective communication between health care providers and patients. A standard bioethical analysis locates SDM as somewhere between the poles of pure paternalism and pure autonomy. We think that this is a good metric, but suggest that, if applied in an overly simplistic way, it may miss more subtle forms of paternalism. Sometimes, doctors attempt to promote autonomy but do so in a way that actually, perhaps unconsciously, undermines respect for the patients. This may occur when doctors, parents, and adolescents shared unmetabolized fear and anger. Such anger can manifest itself in catastrophic and wishful beliefs that hijack the skills necessary for rational decision making.[5]

Doctors, patients, and parents can all become enmeshed in each other's psychodramas without recognizing that such enmeshment is occurring. Such enmeshment can occur even when it seems that doctors are taking an explicitly hands-off, respect-for-autonomy approach. To avoid such enmeshment requires a set of skills that most doctors do not think about and have not been trained to acquire: they must be deeply aware of their own individual values and presumptions. In this case, we wonder if the doctors had deeply held beliefs about whether or not Jorge should undergo a BMT. Had they had bad experiences with such patients in the past? Were they, unconsciously, trying to scare Jorge away, and doing so using techniques that could plausibly appear to be promoting Jorge's autonomy by giving him the brutal facts?

What would an alternative approach look like? Rather than unreflectively sharing the facts with Jorge and his family, the doctors could have tried to create a space for empathic curiosity and listening. If they succeeded, then they would have been in a better position to have explicit discussions about the treatment choices that wouldn't simply terrify Jorge and put his family in an untenable and lonely situation. This case illustrates the problems and suggests ways that communication could be improved.

To reflect on what could have been done better, we will focus on three clinical and research areas: developmental psychology, psychodynamic psychotherapy, and the philosophical foundations of bioethics.

First, developmentally, how can we expect a 13-year-old boy, even one labeled as somewhat "mature," to understand and process information delivered to him this way? How does a young adolescent think about invasive procedures, pain, suffering, isolation, and death itself or even what he might be giving up by not living past 13?

We know that most 13-year-old boys have immature executive function, with insufficient ability to regulate emotions like fear, and difficulties envisioning prospective states.[6] Many such teens and some adults with IDDs are only able to picture two temporal points when they make decisions: now and never. If one cannot envision the future in terms of shades of gray, and if one's thinking is readily hijacked by fear, what does it mean to hear that one's chance of survival 5 years from now is 40%, and only if one goes through a noxious treatment right now? Jorge knew that treatment would cause suffering. Now he also heard that, in spite of that suffering, he was likely to die anyway. All of this was then likely made much worse by the messages that Jorge received from the transplant doctor. Teenagers have a magnified sensory imagination, so although the detailed description of all the pain and suffering associated with the BMT might preoccupy any adult, the odds are high that such details would hijack the attention and imagination of a teenager. It's very possible that Jorge was picturing terrible pain whenever he tried to deliberate about the value of the BMT, perhaps thinking, "die now or go through torture, then die?"

Even for adults, emotions often overwhelm reason. When a person's emotional view of their situation is so vivid and compelling that it becomes impossible to genuinely weigh the risks and benefits, the person is temporarily incapable of the basic deliberation central to decisional capacity.[5] Although we would need to have learned more details to assess Jorge's thinking, we think it is safe to assume that his age and the terrifying details emphasized by the transplant doctor made it likely that he was temporarily hijacked from being capable of meaningful deliberation.

Given these developmental considerations, let us turn to a psychodynamic inquiry into the communicative field between the physicians and Jorge and his family. We assume that the pediatric oncologist and transplant specialist likely knew a great deal about young teenagers and how they process bad news. Still, if the case report is accurate, they discussed bad news with Jorge in a way that did not follow developmental knowledge. Their own emotions may have distorted their thinking process, just the way their communication style distorted Jorge's. From a psychodynamic perspective, the transplant doctor and team may have been protecting themselves from feeling guilty if Jorge died of the BMT. They may have felt guilty about inflicting suffering on the children who went through terrible treatment and then died anyway. Their bluntness might have been an unconscious attempt to minimize the likelihood of experiencing those feelings of guilt. Furthermore, given the prevailing paradigms of bioethics, they could do so in a way that seemed necessary and even admirable. They were not hiding difficult truths, as paternalistic doctors had done in the past. But they were, we suggest, possibly hiding from their own complex emotions.

In addition to these dynamics, the bioethical conclusions drawn rely on philosophical misunderstandings. The doctors believed that their full disclosure of the facts was called for as part of respect for autonomy. The case commentators emphasized Jorge's maturity and stated that his choice to refuse the BMT needed to be respected to respect his autonomy. There are two issues with these judgments. First, even if respect for autonomy was the right goal, Jorge's fear is likely to have hijacked his ability to exercise whatever capacity he had for autonomy (regardless of how mature he was). So, if respect for autonomy was the goal, Jorge's decision could not simply be accepted at face value; rather, there was an obligation to address (and not provoke) his fear and anxiety to make deliberation possible.

Second, respecting Jorge's independent decision about treatment at that time may not have been the right choice even if the goal was to show respect for him as a person. Why? Because this particular decision had to do with how valuable a 40% chance of having a future was to him. In general, 13-year-olds have great difficulty weighing and balancing future-oriented considerations, which are critical to the decision-making task he was facing.[6]

On the other hand, we know that children with chronic diseases often know much more about what it is like living with those diseases and going through noxious treatments than do their parents or physicians. We rightfully do respect their judgments about what they can or cannot tolerate. Jorge's experiential knowledge from having already gone through chemotherapy was crucially important to his decision. He needed to be an active participant in deciding if he felt that he could tolerate the BMT, even if he could not envision the future life that the treatment might help him gain. Thus, Jorge was an ideal candidate for an SDM process, one in which emotional scaffolding from others enabled him to become less afraid and in which he was able to trust and rely on his parents' and physicians' views of his future. His doctors owed Jorge respect. But that required them to respect his actual 13-year-old mind by providing the emotional and intellectual scaffolding by which Jorge could truly engage in a robust process of SDM.

Case 2: A Patient With an Intellectual/ Developmental Disability

Before we continue our discussion of the ethical implications of Jorge's case for SDM, we pause to explore a contrasting case. Though we have identified the ethical problem in this case as the physicians' failure to provide emotional scaffolding, we also acknowledged that in this case, Jorge's physicians may have overestimated his autonomy status, emphasizing his maturity. The contrasting case of R.H. also demonstrates the need for emotional scaffolding. In this case, the doctors underestimated the patient's decisional capacity because of her IDD.

Cases involving adults with IDDs, like the following case, are not typically considered through an SDM lens because of the complex dynamics and legal considerations involved in such decisions. Indeed, the contrasting case of R.H. reveals the difference that an inherently medicolegal approach makes, and the lessons are somewhat distinct from Jorge's case, the primary case considered in this chapter. We use R.H.'s case as a reminder that SDM elements may be an asset in many different situations and as a way to emphasize how the lack of emotional scaffolding, regardless of recognition of autonomy status, weakens and can even undermine respect for persons.

In 1992, R.H. was a 33-year-old woman with Down syndrome.[7] She lived at a residential facility for adults with IDDs where she enjoyed an active social life and worked at a nearby office 4 days a week. Unfortunately, she had chronic pyelonephritis, which progressed to the point that she needed dialysis and an eventual kidney transplant.

Her mother, who was her legal guardian, did not want R.H to have dialysis. She did not think R.H. would have been able to handle the dialysis infusions (because of the needles). R.H.'s mother also worried about what dialysis would require of her, the mother, since she would have to accompany R.H. during each treatment.

The Massachusetts Department of Mental Retardation challenged the mother's refusal of dialysis. They asked the court to appoint a guardian ad litem to assist and be an advocate for R.H. The guardian ad litem agreed with the mother, stating that dialysis was not recommended for R.H.

Crucially, though the probate judge consulted R.H.'s family members, guardian ad litem, and physicians, R.H. was *never* asked what she wanted. Through the lens of R.H.'s diminished autonomy, R.H.'s mother and legal guardian was acting on her behalf and was supposed to be acting in her best interests. Though R.H.'s mother may have felt she was fulfilling her duty as a guardian, as onlookers, we can observe clearly how the assumptions about R.H.'s lack of autonomy had dire consequences for the lack of respect for her as a person.

What did the doctors in the case think? R.H.'s two primary care physicians and the hospital dialysis unit director understood their first ethical obligation to R.H. to be centered on extending her life and stated that dialysis would allow her to live for 10 to 20 years.[8] Judging from past procedures such as blood draws, they felt that R.H. would have been able to tolerate the dialysis and possible future transplant. The dialysis director also testified that she found R.H. to be communicative and able to understand, in a limited way, what was happening to her. The nephrologist, however, agreed with R.H.'s mother and stated that R.H. would not have been able to comprehend the purpose of blood-based dialysis.

Cases like that of R.H. reveal how caregivers and guardians, who are often under enormous strain, may make decisions in the name of beneficence that weaken or destroy any semblance of dignity or respect for the individual's personhood. In this case, R.H.'s personhood was not considered worthy of respect in that she was not asked her opinion on decisions about her own health care.

How could they have approached this differently? By viewing both R.H. *and her mother* as people facing the scary, unknown prospect of painful and laborious treatment or imminent death, they may have been able to provide "emotional scaffolding" when they explained dialysis and subsequent procedures such as a kidney transplant. While in Jorge's case information was provided in a way that was terrifying for the patient, here we have the opposite problem where a complete lack of information and patient input results in a bad outcome. Physicians were caught between the perceived autonomy of R.H.'s mother as her guardian and perceived complete lack of autonomy ascribed to R.H. They did not recognize her as an adult person, did not seek her input, and showed no respect for her. R.H.'s disability status, which is separate from her actual cognitive capacity, is certainly at the root of these approaches to her care.

Respect for Persons as Ethical Focus in Shared Decision Making

The ethical mistake in both cases was to miss crucial ways in which Jorge and R.H. were being disrespected. In Jorge's case, the support for respecting him as a person was not provided under the guise of "respecting his autonomy." In R.H.'s case, reacting to her clearly diminished autonomy, the team failed to even try to respect her as a person. It is not the amount of autonomy that is significant here, but how the lack of attention to respecting persons disallowed emotional scaffolding.

We fail to respect someone as a person when we undermine them psychologically. We can readily see how treating people manipulatively or cruelly can undermine their sense of secure personhood and ongoing-ness in the world (think of how torture or brainwashing undermines narrative personhood). However, it is crucial that we also attend to more subtle or unexpected similar instances of personhood destabilization, particularly in cases of life-threatening medical decision making. For instance, a rupture of personhood can readily occur for a 13-year-old boy facing a terminal diagnosis and horrible treatment options. R.H.'s personhood was ruptured by the absence of communication as she faced a bleak prognosis. The first obligation of doctors, nurses, and social workers is to prevent or help repair such ruptures. It is an ethical imperative for clinicians to be attentive to the emotional context of the information being discussed in SDM. To discuss traumatic facts with a patient without empathic attention to what these facts mean to this particular patient can in and of itself trigger depersonalization. For example, Holocaust survivor Primo Levi recounts how if he were asked to tell about what it was like in a concentration camp and the listener was polite but emotionally neutral, he felt himself to be disappearing.[9]

Returning to Jorge's case, we call attention to the physicians' communication failures as the primary bioethical problem because they failed to respect him as a person. This poor communication has been ignored in commentaries because bioethics sees respectful communication (as opposed to respecting autonomy) as discretionary rather than obligatory. Against this, we emphasize the significance of communication as a mandate for acting in ways that honor ethical principles, also recalling R.H.'s case where the communication never included the patient herself.

In Jorge's case, three crucial things were not done. First, the information was not framed in a way that allowed the patient to process it. Second, the doctors were unaware of their own unconscious motivations. Third, the doctors did not recognize their own limitations and thus failed to bring in people who could have helped the youth and his parents work through and tolerate their otherwise unbearable choice. On this last point, there was a social worker who helped Jorge earlier in his cancer treatment. She was brought in again later in the case after things fell apart, but she was notably absent at the critical moments when the oncologist and then the transplant doctor each delivered the toxic information to Jorge. Just as a burn victim might need to hold a trusted nurse's hand during the most difficult moment of treatment, Jorge likely needed accompaniment during those most traumatic moments, especially because Jorge's parents were just as traumatized by the news. Recognizing and appropriately attending to the parents' role as parents and as persons is another way to respect the persons involved despite the confusion about how to respect patient autonomy. By being sensitive and supportive to all family members involved, as well as by acknowledging the physician's own feelings, respecting persons becomes not a question of whose claims or concerns should trump others, but an ongoing quest to ensure that at every point in a truly horrible scenario, individuals are supported to make the wisest decisions.

Once the damage was done, what should the team have done next? Jorge was owed the scaffolding necessary to restore his sense of ongoing-ness and security as a person. He was owed this regardless of whether he then accepted the BMT. That is, he was owed it out of respect for him as a person, not beneficence.

What are some practical interventions that can provide such scaffolding? Jorge and his parents probably needed more time alone with a trusted therapeutic other like the social worker to ask their questions and address their fears without worrying about the physician's presence or feeling rushed. Note that after Jorge refused treatment, his oncologist did engage in a lengthy meeting with Jorge that included the social worker and others. Presumably the team tried to provide emotional support and a chance for him to express his concerns, but Jorge did not engage. Perhaps it would have helped if his doctor had directly addressed how frightening it must have been to hear such scary messages from the transplant team and himself, but this does not appear to have occurred. But what if none of that helped? What if Jorge had persisted in refusing transplant after all this?

We have already disagreed with the three commentators who say that we ought to accept his decision out of respect for his autonomy because we do not believe that he could exercise autonomy by deliberating (weighing and balancing both sides) in the case of this particular decision. When we cannot respect the autonomy of a minor or person who has not been legally granted autonomy, we shift some weight to our obligation to serve their best interests. But at the same time, we have argued that we still owe Jorge respect as a person.

How does this actually translate into action? Such cases involve a fundamental tension between the desire to respect Jorge as a person and the desire to do what is best for him. Such tensions also arise in cases where we restrain an actively suicidal but apparently competent patient. Such restraint itself is not an expression of respect for the patient as a person; it is rooted purely in beneficence.

Being clear on the difference between the obligations from beneficence and those from respect for persons keeps us attentive to the moral obligations that persist when we must infringe on a person's rights to promote their best interests. In Jorge's case, given that he is only 13, there is a strong argument for allowing beneficence to outweigh, but not eliminate, the obligation to respect his wishes. That argument is that he is not yet responsible for his own life in the way an adult is. Instead, his parents and his doctors are strongly responsible for his well-being.

Children require support not only for the practical aspects of life but also for their emotional, social, and educational needs. Thus, Ross,[10] Salter,[7] and others have shown that the issue of decisional *responsibility* for adolescents is important and distinct from the issue of decisional capacity. In their work, the emphasis is on parental authority for such decisions, given that parents are responsible for shepherding adolescents into adulthood. Although we agree with their arguments, our focus is not on parents per se but on how the fact that children require physical, emotional, and social resources to have a decent life trajectory creates a societal responsibility to protect their best interests. Usually, parents appropriately take on much of this responsibility, as Jorge's parents did. In this case, his parents and medical team might have, as a last resort, decided to override Jorge's decision (out of beneficence, not respect). In that case, they should convey to Jorge that they are overriding him but will defer to him for the smaller decisions about the circumstances of his undergoing the BMT, when to return home and to school, etc.

It is possible, even likely, that Jorge would have ultimately accepted this and felt adequately safe and respected and loved. Thirteen-year-olds often feel safer when their more dangerous choices are overridden. Thus, the balancing of respect and beneficence would lean toward beneficence, but some respect for him as a person would remain. Alternatively, in the worst-case scenario, telling him that he will have the transplant could trigger some lasting negative reaction on his part. Unfortunately, a BMT differs from a one-time surgery or even 72-hour psychiatric hold in that it can involve months of suffering. If Jorge were to experience this suffering as forced on him, he could experience an ongoing state of terror akin to what people experience when they are prisoners subject to torture, and it would be difficult to justify imposing this on him even for his long-term best interests. Possibly we could shift his fear level by promising (truthfully) that if he could not tolerate the situation after the procedure and there was no other way of alleviating his suffering, he could be given comfort measures only and enabled to pass away quickly rather than stay in a prolonged state of involuntary suffering. This is of course an ethically fraught situation, but it does seem unjustifiable to force him to go through months of fear and suffering against his will.

Insights from Jorge's case may not be relevant to all situations in which adolescents face difficult decisions. Prognosis, the burdens of therapies, and the urgency of the decision could all affect how respectful communication can best be structured to provide a supportive and safe environment for both the adolescent and the family. Even more importantly, however, creating such a space is necessary even when there does not appear to be disagreement with a recommended plan. Jorge's refusal of the transplant made his fears apparent to the medical team; other patients who do not object may be suffering in silence.

Conclusions

In this chapter, we highlighted two cases from the 1990s. In the first case, the medical team was hijacked by unconscious emotional projections and the bioethics reviewers were stymied by a need-lessly narrow view of their obligation to respect autonomy. In the second, an adult with IDD was ignored and disrespected because her caregivers did not see her as a person worthy of respect.

Both cases are quite contemporary insofar as physicians continue to be unreflective of the role of their own unconscious emotions in how they frame treatment options for seriously ill adolescents, for adults with IDDs, and for their families. This inadvertent emotional "sharing" needs to be reflected upon now as we try to build a solid foundation for new models of SDM. Although some might argue that such attention to the emotional underpinnings of difficult decisions is not a component of the process of SDM, we would argue that it is impossible to approach SDM without it. For physicians with seriously ill patients, communicating in ways that create security and trust is not optional. Before we bring in new models of SDM, we need to ensure that doctors know how to create the foundational conditions for good communication. For physicians providing care for adults with IDDs, this means under-standing how a disability status does not preclude respect and un-derstanding the often-enmeshed relationship between caregivers and guardians and individuals with IDDs. For pediatricians, this requires knowing enough about how adolescents process cognitive, affective, and sensory information to avoid traumatizing their patients; knowing enough about the doctor's own fears not to project them onto the patient; and providing the supportive others who can help the teenager tolerate and process information that is otherwise intolerable. Failing to do so can lead to tragic outcomes.

References

1. Kon AA. The shared decision-making continuum. *JAMA*. 2010;304(8): 903–904.
2. Halpern J. The therapeutic effects of empathy in healthcare. 2017. Available at: http://emotionresearcher.com/the-therapeutic-effects-of-empathy-in-healthcare/. Accessed May 21, 2018.
3. Stein MT, Wells R, Stephenson S, Schneiderman LJ. Decision making about medical care in an adolescent with a life-threatening illness. *Pediatrics*. 2001;107(Suppl 1):979–982.
4. Klugman C. Cassandra C: right to refuse treatment or protecting a minor. Available at: www. bioethics.net/2015/01/cassandra-c-right-to-refuse-treatment-or-protecting-a-minor/. Accessed May 21, 2018.
5. Halpern J. When concretized emotion-belief complexes derail decision-making capacity. *Bioethics*. 2012;26(2):108–116.
6. Salter EK. Conflating capacity & authority: why we're asking the wrong question in the adolescent decision-making debate. *Hastings Cent Rep*. 2017;47(1):32–41.
7. Miller EC. Listening to the disabled: end-of-life medical decision making and the never competent. *Fordham L. Rev.* 2005;74:2889.
8. Davis SM. In re RH. *Issues L. & Med.* 1994;10:229.
9. Halpern J. Empathy and patient-physician conflicts. *J Gen Intern Med*. 2007;22(5):696–700.
10. Ross LF. Against the tide: arguments against respecting a minor's refusal of efficacious life-saving treatment. *Camb Q Healthc Ethics*. 2009;18(3):302–315; discussion 315–322.

6

Serious Pediatric Illness

A Spectrum of Clinician Directiveness in Collaborative Decision Making

Jonna D. Clark, Mithya Lewis-Newby, Alexander A. Kon, and Wynne Morrison

Evolution of Clinician-Patient Decision-Making Models in Western Medicine

Over the past two decades, shared decision making (SDM) has become the recommended approach to medical decision making, especially in serious illness.[1-3] SDM is often viewed as a middle ground between two ends of a spectrum: parentalism (aka paternalism), where clinicians make decisions they believe are in the best interests of their patients without patient input, and a model based on respect for patient autonomy, where patients are expected to choose among several possible therapeutic options, often without explicit guidance from clinicians. Both of these models are flawed. Parentalism does not promote respect for patient and family autonomy, even though patients have the right to make their own decisions about their health. On the other hand, prioritizing respect for patient autonomy, where clinicians offer a list of neutral options without explicit guidance or recommendations, can lead patients and families to feel abandoned, overwhelmed, and confused, resulting in decisions that may not be in the best interest of the patient.

To prevent these challenges, SDM creates an ideal model, where the medical expertise of the clinician and the preferences and values of the patient and family are aligned, resulting in the best decision for the patient. However, operationalization of SDM can be difficult, especially in pediatrics, where there are not clear guidelines on balancing limitations of parental authority and incorporating the role of the vulnerable child.[5,6] Furthermore, a unified definition of SDM remains under discussion.

Some organizations endorse a model where the "sharing" in the model is "equal," while other organizations use a definition that is more flexible and encourage adaptation of the model to the clinical context and unique circumstances surrounding the decision.[2,7] For the purpose of this chapter, SDM is defined as "a collaborative process that allows patients, their surrogates, and clinicians to make health care decisions together, taking into account the best scientific evidence available, as well as the patient's values, goals, and preferences."[2] The terminology of "family" is used to refer to anyone who provides support for the child and plays a role in medical decision making, whether or not they are directly related to the patient or have legal decision-making rights. "Parents" is used to represent the legal guardians, and "clinician" is used to refer to any health care professional who assists the family with making medical decisions for the child.

Collaborative Decision Making Versus Shared Decision Making

We favor the term "collaborative decision making" (CDM) as an evolution from the term "shared decision making" for the following three reasons. First, the term "*shared* decision making" can be interpreted as that decisions are *equally* shared. However, not all medical decisions allow for *equal* sharing, nor is *equal sharing* always desired by patients and families. Rather, there is a spectrum along which clinicians may be more or less directive in the decision-making process. The degree of clinician directiveness is influenced by myriad factors, which we explore later in this chapter.[8-12] Furthermore, the degree of clinician directiveness evolves and changes depending on the clinical and family context. Second, most medical decisions, even urgent ones, are commonly made over a series of conversations using a collaborative process over time, where there is an "exchange of information and knowledge with *joint* exploration of values to arrive at a decision that is in the best interest of the child and minimizes harm."[11] Third, "collaboration," more so than "sharing," implies a cooperative partnership, built on trust, where the stakeholders work together as a team to accomplish a specified goal.

Collaborative Decision Making in Pediatric Patients

The *pediatric* setting adds complexity to medical decision making.[13,14] The relationship between a clinician, family, and child differs in important ways from the relationship between a clinician and an autonomous adult or their surrogate. Autonomous adults have a lot of latitude to make medical choices that align best with their own values. Similarly, surrogates for adults are tasked with making decisions consistent with the prior expressed wishes of the patient using substituted judgment. Children, on the other hand, often do not participate in medical decisions at the same level as adults, and there is a wide range of participation depending on age and development. Most children have short life experiences and do not have established values or long-term goals, and therefore have limited ability to propose what they would want in certain circumstances. In pediatrics, the "best interest standard" is used, where decisions by parents and clinicians are made based on their perceptions of what is in the best interest of the child. Most often clinicians and families are aligned in "best interest" decision making. However, while parents generally have the authority to make decisions for their children, this authority is not absolute. Parents are not allowed to make decisions where the harm greatly outweighs the potential benefit, and clinicians need not offer interventions that are outside the boundaries of accepted medical practice or interventions they believe would be unreasonable.[14,15]

Medical decision making in pediatric *serious illness* also increases complexity. Decisions are often high stakes, involving life-and-death consequences. Occasionally, in serious pediatric illness, decision-making stakeholders may have different value-based opinions about which decision is best for the child. Clinicians often have their own value-based opinions. Additionally, families have a range of desire and comfort with making decisions.[8] The high-stakes nature of decisions in serious pediatric illness often leads to an emotionally intense environment, where families may struggle to make decisions if they feel overwhelmed or burdened. When the decision may impact living versus dying, some parents may prioritize perceived quality of life for their child and worry about prolonged suffering. Others may perceive limiting life-sustaining therapies, even in the face of very low likelihood of survival, as "giving up" on their child, which may be considered the ultimate harm.[16,17]

Furthermore, sometimes decisions are more urgent than others and need to be made within a short time frame. When there is greater urgency, families may feel the need to defer decisions to clinicians, who have greater medical expertise. Since survivors of serious illness may have significant morbidity, impacting functional status and quality of life, families may struggle to assess the degree to which their child is suffering and lack a clear understanding of how their quality of life may be impacted.[18]

Finally, medical decisions for serious illness often require a high level of technical expertise or advanced medical knowledge. While some families may have extensive experience in the medical environment, others may enter with limited health literacy. Under these circumstances, families may need additional time and guidance to understand the nuances in the decisions associated with the highly technical environment.

Empirical Evidence Supporting Collaborative Decision Making

Several studies show that the implementation of specific aspects of SDM improves patient and family satisfaction and reduces decisional regret.[4,19] When families were informed about options, they felt more certain about their decision, understood the risks and benefits, and felt more supported to make the decision. Parents have less emotional conflict and less regret when physicians explore the family's values to help them reach decisions.[20] Parents even have more success getting access to health care services when doctors work with them to make decisions.[21,22]

The Spectrum of Clinician Directiveness

CDM can be applied in any clinical circumstance, but flexibility and adaptation of the model to each individual situation and context are necessary. In all contexts, CDM has several key components.[2,22,23] These include:

1. Establishment of trust between clinician and family
2. Recognition that medical decision making is usually a process that spans multiple conversations
3. Open, empathetic, nonjudgmental communication between clinician and family
4. Acknowledgment of the high level of emotion (family and clinicians) involved in complex decisions

5. Awareness that prognostic uncertainty may make decision making more complex

The development of a trusting partnership between the clinician, family, and, when appropriate, the child is essential in CDM. Patients' values and preferences are not developed in isolation. Rather, they are defined and shaped by others in trusting relationships.[24] In such relationships, the family shares their values and goals for the child with the clinician. The clinician serves as a special guide, sharing medical information using a variety of means, exploring family values under the specific circumstances, and assisting with deliberation. Together, the clinician and the family come to the best decision possible.[26] Clinician communication skills, empathy, and emotional intelligence are necessary to develop a connection with the family.[27,28] Eliciting the family's understanding of the clinical situation and values can sometimes be very difficult, especially if a trusting partnership has not been developed.[29] Often, interdisciplinary teamwork may be beneficial. In many cases, the focus is not on the information itself but, instead, on the emotions and values that are shared among patients, family members, and clinicians. These are essential to the mutual understanding that optimizes decision making.[24,25]

Families often make decisions that are influenced by a combination of internal and external factors. External values may come from social media or support groups, prior experiences, the need to take care of someone else's psychological needs or "protect" other family members, and the family's ability to process complex information and ambiguity.[17,24] Internal factors include the family's focus on the child's suffering and quality of life.[17] When faced with difficult decisions under circumstances that are novel and extremely stressful, family preferences may be vague, unstable, or uninformed.[24] Envisioning the child's future, and the family's future, may be difficult. Although most families adapt to the "new normal" of raising a child with a disability, some do not.[30]

Decision making can be an evolving process. The clinician engages in a model of relationship that is interactional rather than transactional, with a mindset of curiosity and consensus rather than negotiation and consent, and with a deep sense of awareness and empathy rather than concreteness and lack of personal connection.[24] In general, when making complex decisions, families express the need to know that their child is being treated medically, that the best care possible is being provided, and they need to feel hopeful.[31]

Spectrum of Clinician Directiveness Within Clinical Decision Making

Flexibility and adaptation to different circumstances result in a spectrum of clinician directiveness in the CDM process.[10] Titrating clinician directiveness within the fluidity of the clinician-family-patient partnership is the "art" of CDM. The clinician has an ethical obligation to explore, develop, and understand the perspective and values of the patient and family under the new set of circumstances that accompany serious illness. The clinician can help the family to see how those values may guide choices among the available medical options.[11,32] However, clinicians need to retain insight and perspective into how their own values and biases may influence their recommendations.[33-39] Within this partnership of CDM, we describe a model of four general levels of clinician directiveness along a spectrum to help guide the clinician.[10]

Low: Some families prefer to make decisions relatively independently. For such families, the clinician can present the range of appropriate medical choices and explain how each of these options may "play out" for the individual child relative to the family's values. This is similar to an "informed" model, where the clinician provides information and allows the family to decide.[7] Often, different families will make different decisions under the same set of circumstances. The clinician should provide ongoing support to the family and help them explore their values.

Moderate: Some families ask for additional guidance. Then, the clinician may make a stronger recommendation, based on their assessment of the child's interest and on their understanding of the family's values and goals. This recommendation may be presented as a "default" option and framed in such a way that the family hears the option as the recommended option.[40,41] Other options should also be explained in a way that helps the family understand that they can make the decision that best aligns with their values and goals without judgment from the clinician.

High: Sometimes, the clinician may feel strongly that certain choices are more likely to prevent additional harm or lead to greater benefit. Some families may wish to cede decision-making authority to the clinician. This deference may stem from a desire to avoid an extremely emotionally laden decision (e.g., compassionate extubation or forgoing attempted resuscitation) or be based on a cultural value of deferring difficult medical decisions to "authority." As with all aspects of CDM, for this model to be effective, a trusting partnership between the clinician and family is required. The family needs to feel that their child is deeply cared for and is receiving the highest quality of medical care, and that all decisions are made in the best interest of the child. This model has been described as "informed nondissent."[42-45] It can be effective for families that express a preference toward greater directiveness and guidance from the clinician.[46,47]

Near complete: Often this approach is used when there are few or only one appropriate medical option. While benefit and burden are often subjective and value laden, there are certain circumstances in medicine when few choices exist. For example, treating a previously healthy child with septic shock with antibiotics is necessary based on the high likelihood of a good outcome, and parental authority to refuse antibiotics is limited.[14] Under these circumstances, the clinician will be very directive in guiding medical care. Alternatively, when a child with leukemia following a third bone marrow transplant suffers from multiorgan system failure due to disseminated fungus and relapsed leukemia, a clinician may be directive in making the decision not to place the child on extracorporeal life support. Under these circumstances, the clinician should not offer choices that are not medically indicated as determined by team consensus. We suggest that therapies be defined as "not medically indicated" if it they are not expected to provide any physiological benefit.[15] We recognize that there are no universally accepted definitions of the term "not medically indicated."

Using a more directive approach does not necessarily mean that disputes between clinicians and families will be avoided, especially when decisions are high stakes in an extremely emotional environment. On the contrary, if directive approaches are used without first establishing a sense of respectful and trusting partnership, this approach can lead to an escalation in conflict. However, by building a trusting partnership and assuring families that the child is deeply cared about as an individual person, families can often feel supported under these tragic circumstances. Sometimes, in extreme cases, even under the best attempts to build a relationship, disputes may occur. For these situations, referring to guidance on how to resolve these disputes can be helpful.[15,48]

Internal and External Influences on the Degree of Clinician Directiveness

Determining the appropriate level of clinician directiveness is often a complex and dynamic process. The degree of clinician directiveness is often influenced by four factors: the characteristics of the decision, the specifics of the disease and treatment, the nature of the collaborative decision-making team, and external influences, such as the institution and society.[10]

Decision-Related Characteristics

Characteristics related to the type of decision are important to consider. In pediatric serious illness, some decisions need to be made urgently, whereas others allow for more time. Feeling pressured by an urgent decision, a family may choose to cede the decision to a clinician, whereas a nonurgent decision may allow the family to gain a better understanding of the nuances of the decision prior to making a decision. Furthermore, decisions in serious illness often have life-or-death consequences or, if death is not likely, may result in substantial morbidity. Under these circumstances, a family may feel like there is no choice, as death is the ultimate harm to their child.[16] Other times, a family may feel overwhelmed by the emotional burden of the decision due to the high-stakes nature and ask the clinician to guide or even make the decision, especially if the decision results in the death of their child. Finally, for decisions that are highly technical, a family may defer to the expertise of the clinician, whereas for decisions that are more value or preference based, a clinician may offer the family to take greater responsibility for the decision. However, assumptions should be avoided, as not all families prefer to cede technical decisions to clinicians, nor should all families be expected to take full responsibility for value-based decisions.

Disease- and Treatment-Related Characteristics

The prognosis, degree of prognostic certainty, potential morbidities, and time course of the disease are also important factors to consider when titrating the degree of clinician directiveness. Disease processes with greater prognostic certainty may lend to an approach where clinicians take more responsibility for a decision, acknowledging there is greater certainty in outcome with a standard treatment or intervention. On the other hand, for diseases where there is greater prognostic uncertainty, or for disease processes that are prolonged with significant morbidity, families may take more responsibility for the decision. Of note, sometimes families prefer to take responsibility for the decision but first seek permission from the clinician to make the decision, especially when the decision involves shifting goals of care from aggressive life-saving therapies to comfort care measures. Navigating these complex circumstances can be difficult, and using collaborative and empathetic communication can be highly beneficial.

The type of treatment may also impact the clinician degree of directiveness in decision making. Whether the treatment or intervention is standard of care or experimental often impacts whether a clinician is more or less directive with a family. If the standard of care has a high likelihood of success with low risk, the clinician likely will be more directive, whereas if the treatment or intervention is experimental or high risk, the clinician may offer the family to play a greater role in the decision.

Characteristics of the Collaborative Decision-Making Team

CDM occurs within the context of the patient, family, and clinician. During pediatric serious illness, families often enter into the clinical setting carrying their own narrative, prior experiences, cultural backgrounds, and value systems. While all of these factors influence what decision is made, these factors also contribute to how a decision is made. For some families with limited exposure to the health care system, they may be more deferential to the expertise of the medical team, whereas families with greater experience may want to take responsibility for all decisions. Based on their cultural background, some families may cede to a faith or community leader. Understanding the context from which the family comes and what their preferences are in regard to their preferred role in decision making is crucial in determining how directive a clinician should be in decision making. Furthermore, clinicians also have their own medical expertise, values, biases, and comfort level in being directive with patients and families. Some clinicians feel very uncomfortable making complex decisions for families, whereas others prefer to make the decisions for families. In addition, clinicians also have ethical and legal obligations that might guide a decision. Introspective reflection of biases and preferences, maintaining curiosity, and collaboration with colleagues can help guide clinicians in how to adjust their directiveness with families.

Extrinsic Influences

Institutional and societal values also impact how decisions are made. Institutions have prior experiences and perspectives on pediatric serious illness, imbedded biases and preferences, power dynamics, policies, and legal obligations. These factors also impact how families are approached when faced with pediatric serious illnesses. Institutional policy may guide clinicians in being very directive regarding not offering life-sustaining therapies that have a very low chance of benefit. Furthermore, institutions exist within societies that also have values, biases, and judicial regulations. In the United States, we might approach SDM differently than in a country with socialized medicine that may have tight restrictions on expensive interventions, or a country where parentalism is the unified approach to making decisions. Finally, sometimes clinicians prefer to be more directive when they have concerns regarding how a decision might impact the care of other children or the allocation of scarce resources. In other rare circumstances, there may be concerns about the impact of a decision on public health. Careful analyses of these influences is important to create transparency regarding how directive clinicians may be in decision making in pediatric serious illness.

Maintaining flexibility in clinician directiveness may reduce two serious risks: (1) the clinician is so directive that the family does not feel heard or cared about, and (2) the clinician is so nondirective that the family feels abandoned and forced to make a difficult decision without support and guidance.[10]

Barriers and Enablers to Optimizing Collaborative Decision Making

While the ideal of CDM is appealing, the practical implementation may be challenging. Multiple barriers exist.[49] High staff turnover through shift work and frequent clinical team rotations negatively impacts the clinical team's ability to build trusting partnerships with families. Patients with serious illness are often hospitalized in busy units; due to other clinical needs, time for conversations may be limited between clinicians and families. Clinical teams are complex and often include multiple types of professionals, subspecialists, and trainees, many of whom have a relationship with the family. Communication from different team members sometimes may be perceived as incongruous. The physical environment in the hospital setting may disrupt CDM if it contributes to family discomfort. Families may be disconcerted by the unfamiliar setting, sterile and loud environment, lack of sleep space, and limited visiting hours.[50] Finally, despite the attempt to eliminate power differentials with families, the hospital setting automatically defers power to clinicians by sheer familiarity with the environment.[49,50]

Several recommendations may help foster CDM. First, using an adaptable and flexible approach, incorporating active listening, curiosity, and clinical humility are essential to discern and understand a family's preferences, values, priorities, and needs. The needs and preferences of families may change for different decisions, at different times, and with different clinicians. Frequent "check-backs" with families can be helpful to ensure that there is clarity in understanding.

Second, trying to maintain clinician continuity will be helpful in creating collaborative partnerships.[49] Employing a "continuity attending physician" model may help families feel more connected to a single clinician. Building team consensus regarding potentially inappropriate interventions can help maintain trust and prevent decisions based merely on individual clinician value judgments.

Third, recognize that making difficult decisions is a time-consuming process. "Planting seeds" for what may happen and what decisions might need to be made in the future helps families navigate their journeys.[51]

Finally, using a multidisciplinary approach can be beneficial. Early palliative care consultation may enable families to more deeply explore their values, goals, and hopes to help guide difficult decisions. Spiritual care leaders and cultural navigators may be an additional layer of support that may reduce additional emotional distress related to cultural or faith-based differences or help families navigate the complex Western medical system. Health care ethics consultation may be important to help families when conflict arises or when there are questions about the feasibility of certain options.

Conclusions

Collaborative medical decision making in serious pediatric illness is a process that engages the family and clinician in a trusting partnership to make the best possible decision, aligning the clinician's medical expertise with the values, preferences, and wishes of the family. The model requires a trusting partnership between the clinician and family, open and nonjudgmental dialogue, acknowledgment of the emotional intensity of the decision, and recognition that decisions are made as a process over time. Within this model, the degree to which the clinician is directive in providing medical guidance lies along a spectrum, ranging from low to moderate to high to near complete. Determining the appropriate degree of clinician directiveness depends on myriad characteristics related to the decision, diagnosis and treatment, family and clinician, and institution and society. Maintaining flexibility and adaptability and titrating the degree of clinician directiveness based on the context are essential to providing optimal support to families who face difficult decisions in pediatric serious illness. Often, with this approach, families will not feel abandoned and may experience a greater sense of support, have less decisional regret, and know that their child is deeply cared about and receiving the best medical care possible.

References

1. Barry MJ, Edgman-Levitan S. Shared decision making–pinnacle of patient-centered care. *N Engl J Med*. 2012;366(9):780–781.
2. Kon AA, Davidson JE, Morrison W, Danis M, White DB; American College of Critical Care Medicine; American Thoracic Society. Shared decision making in ICUs: an American College of Critical Care Medicine and American Thoracic Society policy statement. *Crit Care Med*. 2016;44(1):188–201.
3. Kon A, Morrison W. Shared decision making in pediatric practice: a broad view. *Pediatrics*. 2018;142(s3):s129–s130.
4. Wyatt KD, List B, Brinkman W, et al. Shared decision making in pediatrics: a systematic review and meta-analysis. *Acad Pediatr*. 2015;15(6):573–583.
5. Opel DJ. A push for progress with shared decision-making in pediatrics. *Pediatrics*. 2017;139(2):1–3.
6. Opel DJ. A 4-step framework for shared decision making in pediatrics. *Pediatrics*. 2018;142(s3):s149–s156.
7. Charles C, Whelan T, Gafni A. What do we mean by partnership in making decisions about treatment? *BMJ*. 1999;319(7212):780–782.
8. Benbassat J, Pilpel D, Tidhar M. Patients' preferences for participation in clinical decision making: a review of published surveys. *Behav Med*. 1998;24(2):81–88.
9. Kon AA. The shared decision-making continuum. *JAMA*. 2010; 304(8):903–904.

10. Morrison W, Clark J, Lewis-Newby M, Kon A. Titrating clinician directiveness in serious pediatric illness. *Pediatrics.* 2018;142:s178–s186.
11. Moyihan KM, Jansen M, Liaw S-N, Alexander PMA, Truog R. An ethical claim for providing recommendations in pediatric intensive care. *PCCM.* 2018;19:e433–e437.
12. Weiss EM, Barg FK, Cook N, Black E, Joffe S. Parental decision-making preferences in neonatal intensive care. *J Pediatr.* 2016;179:36–41.
13. Baines P. Medical ethics for children: applying the four principles to paediatrics. *J Med Ethics.* 2008;34(3):141–145.
14. Diekema DS. Parental refusals of medical treatment: the harm principle as threshold for state intervention. *Theor Med Bioeth.* 2004;25(4):243–264.
15. Bosslet GT, Pope TM, Rubenfeld GD, et al. An official ATS/AACN/ACCP/ESICM/SCCM policy statement: responding to requests for potentially inappropriate treatments in intensive care units. *Am J Respir Crit Care Med.* 2015;191(11):1318–1330.
16. Curley MA, Meyer EC. Parental experience of highly technical therapy: survivors and nonsurvivors of extracorporeal membrane oxygenation support. *PCCM.* 2003;4:214–219.
17. Zaal-Schuller IH, de Vos MA, Ewals FVPM, vanGoudoever JB, Willems DL. End-of-life decision-making for children with severe developmental disabilities: the parental perspective. *Res Dev Disabil.* 2016;49–50:235–246.
18. Gorgos A, Ghosh S, Payot A. A shared vision of quality of life: partnering decision-making to understand families' realities. *Paediatr Respir Rev.* 2019;29:14–18.
19. Boland L, Kryworuchko J, Saarimaki A, Lawson ML. Parental decision making involvement and decisional conflict: a descriptive study. *BMC Pediatr.* 2017;17(146):1–8.
20. Lipstein EA, Lovell DJ, Denson LA, et al. High levels of decisional conflict and decision regret when making decisions about biologics. *J Pediatr Gastroenterol Nutr.* 2016;63:e176–e181.
21. Jolles MP, Lee P-J, Javier JR. Shared decision making and parental experiences with health services to meet their child's special health care needs: racial and ethnic disparities. *Patient Educ Couns.* 2018;101:1753–1760.
22. Durand MA, Dolan H, Bravo P, Mann M, Bunn F, Elwyn G. Do interventions designed to support shared decision making reduce health inequalities? A systematic review and meta-analysis. *PLoS One.* 2014;9(4):1–13.
23. Feudtner C. Collaborative communication in pediatric palliative care: a foundation for problem-solving and decision-making. *Pediatr Clin North Am.* 2007;54(5):583–607.
24. Epstein RM, Street RL. Shared mind: communication, decision making, and autonomy in serious illness. *Ann Fam Med.* 2011;9:454–461.

25. Azoulay E, Chaize M, Kentish-Barnes N. Involvement of ICU families in decisions: fine-tuning the partnership. *Ann Intensive Care.* 2014;4(37):1–10.

26. Austin CA, Mohottige D, Sudore RL, Smith AK, Hanson LC. Tools to promote shared decision making in serious illness: a systematic review. *JAMA Int Med.* 2015;175(7):1213–1221.

27. Madrigal VN, Patterson Kelly K. Supporting family decision-making for a child who is seriously ill: creating synchrony and connection. *Pediatrics.* 2018;142(s3):s170–s177.

28. Morrison W, Madrigal V. "My way or the highway" versus "whatever the family wants": intensivists reject both extremes. *Pediatr Crit Care Med.* 2012;13:612–613.

29. Smith MA, Clayman ML, Frader J, et al. A descriptive study of decision-making conversations during pediatric intensive care unit family conferences. *J Palliat Med.* 2018;21(9):1290–1299.

30. Albrecht G, Devlieger P. The disability paradox: high quality of life against all odds. *Soc Sci Med.* 1999;48:977–988.

31. Kirschbaum MS. Needs of parents of critically ill children. *Dimens Crit Care Nurs.* 1990;9:344–352.

32. Hill DL, Miller V, Walter JK, et al. Regoaling: a conceptual model of how parents of children with serious illness change medical care goals. *BMC Palliat Care.* 2014;13(1):9.

33. Alfandre D. Clinical recommendations in medical practice: a proposed framework to reduce bias and improve the quality of medical decisions. *J Clin Ethics.* 2016;27:21–27.

34. Racine E, Bell E, Farlow B, et al. The ouR-HOPE approach for ethics and communication about neonatal neurological injury. *Dev Med Child Neurol.* 2017;59:125–135.

35. Sprung CL, Maia P, Bulow HH, et al.; Ethicus Study Group. The importance of religious affiliation and culture on end-of-life decisions in European intensive care units. *Intensive Care Med.* 2007;33(10):1732–1739.

36. Truog RD. "Doctor, if this were your child, what would you do?" *Pediatrics.* 1999;103(1):153–154.

37. Kon AA. Answering the question: "Doctor, if this were your child, what would you do?" *Pediatrics.* 2006;118(1):393–397.

38. Ross LF. Why "doctor, if this were your child, what would you do?" deserves an answer. *J Clin Ethics.* 2003;14(1–2):59–62.

39. Halpern J. Responding to the need behind the question "Doctor, if this were your child, what would you do?" *J Clin Ethics.* 2003;14(1–2):71–78.

40. Halpern SD, Ubel PA, Asch DA. Harnessing the power of default options to improve health care. *N Engl J Med.* 2007;357(13):1340–1344.

41. Feudtner C, Munson D, Morrison W. Framing permission for halting or continuing life-extending therapies. *Virtual Mentor.* 2008;10(8):506–510.

42. Curtis JR, Burt RA. Point: the ethics of unilateral "do not resuscitate" orders: the role of "informed assent." *Chest.* 2007;132(3):748–751.
43. Curtis JR. The use of informed assent in withholding cardiopulmonary resuscitation in the ICU. *Virtual Mentor.* 2012;14(7):545–550.
44. Kon AA. Informed nondissent rather than informed assent. *Chest.* 2008;133(1):320–321.
45. Kon AA. Informed non-dissent: a better option than slow codes when families cannot bear to say "Let her die." *Am J Bioethics.* 2011;11(11):22–23.
46. Madrigal VN, Carroll KW, Hexem KR, Faerber JA, Morrison WE, Feudtner C. Parental decision-making preferences in the pediatric intensive care unit. *Crit Care Med.* 2012;40(10):2876–2882.
47. Weiss EM, Xie D, Cook N, Coughlin K, Joffe S. Characteristics associated with preferences for parent-centered decision making in neonatal intensive care. *JAMA Pediatr.* 2018;172(5):461–468.
48. Kon AA, Shepard EK, Sederstrom NO, et al. Defining futile and potentially inappropriate interventions: a policy statement from the society of critical care medicine ethics committee. *Crit Care Med.* 2016;44(9):1769–1774.
49. Boland L, Graham ID, Legare F, et al. Barriers and facilitators of pediatric shared decision-making: a systematic review. *Implement Sci.* 2019;14(7):1–25.
50. MacDonald ME, Liben S, Carnevale FA, et al. An office or a bedroom? Challenges for family centered care in the pediatric intensive care unit. *J Child Health Care.* 2012;16(3):237–249.
51. Brown A, Clark J. A parent's journey: incorporating principles of palliative care into practice for children with chronic neurologic diseases. *Semin Pediatr Neurol.* 2015;22:159–165.
52. October TW, Fisher KR, Feudtner C, Hinds PS. The parent perspective: "being a good parent" when making critical decisions in the PICU. *Pediatr Crit Care Med.* 2014;15(4):291–298.
53. Hinds PS, Oakes LL, Hicks J, et al. "Trying to be a good parent" as defined by interviews with parents who made phase I, terminal care, and resuscitation decisions for their children. *J Clin Oncol.* 2009;27(35):5979–5985.

7

A Pragmatic Guide to Shared Decision Making

A Justification and Concrete Steps

Jennifer K. Walter and Alexander G. Fiks

There has been inadequate penetrance of shared decision making (SDM) into clinical practice.[1-6] In this chapter, we begin by outlining some of the primary barriers that limit SDM implementation and the potential benefits of health system–level solutions. Then, using the case of an adolescent with advanced cancer, we articulate the pragmatic skills needed to engage in SDM. To increase the dissemination of SDM, patients (and/or their parents) need to be involved,[7,8] and barriers to SDM[9] must be identified and confronted. Clinician comfort with SDM approaches represents one key step in achieving this goal.

Challenges to Shared Decision-Making Implementation

Three factors contribute to the limited penetrance of SDM in clinical practice: (1) clinicians' beliefs that their patients do not want to participate in SDM or that SDM is inappropriate given the options available, (2) a lack of pragmatic guidance on how to conduct SDM, and (3) clinicians' beliefs that SDM is too time-consuming and therefore unfeasible. We will briefly explore some of the data dispelling the first claim and then offer techniques to reduce the second and third concerns.

Misperception That Shared Decision Making Is Not Desired by Patients

According to a systematic review of the adult literature, physicians attribute their lack of use of SDM to patients' preferences and the inapplicability of SDM to their practice population.[5,10] Doctors perceive their role to be one of convincing rather than engaging families in a shared process of decision making.[11] However, physicians may misjudge their patients' desire for active involvement.[12-15] A systematic review of pediatric SDM found an agreement by both the physician and family that they want to have an SDM discussion to be a facilitator of SDM.[16] Patients are different. Some patients with lower health literacy may rely more heavily on the physician's assessment of the medical facts. But they too still want their values to drive choices. Raising a decision as eligible for SDM often depends on the clinical team. Patients may fail to have discussions focused on SDM for fear of being labeled "difficult."[17]

Limited Pragmatic Guidance on How to Operationalize Shared Decision Making

Clinicians who want to use an SDM process may not have the skills needed to operationalize SDM.[18] Limited pragmatic advice is available regarding which steps physicians should take in conversations. Research on SDM has largely focused on the analysis of decision aids. It rarely includes a protocol for how physicians should use the decision aid.[19]

Several teachable communication skills are essential for high-quality SDM.[20] Physicians must be prepared to handle the strong patient and family emotions that arise in discussions about difficult choices.[16] Doctors may be unsure of when or how to elicit patient and family preferences and values.[16] If clinicians are unskilled in eliciting families' values, they are much more likely to offer only one option or strongly emphasize the physician's preferred option.[16] Another potential barrier is communicating clearly with individuals who have low health literacy.[16] Such people lack "the capacity to obtain, process, and understand basic health information."[21,22] Parents with low health literacy defer more to their child's doctor's knowledge in decision making.[9] Parents with higher health literacy scores are more likely to indicate that they want more control over the decision-making process.[23]

One challenge specific to pediatric SDM is determining the role that the patient can play and how to engage them in the conversation. Involving patients with a range of developmental skills is not as simple as relying upon age-based communication recommendations. Adolescents have unique emotional needs. Ignoring those needs may lead to miscommunication and bad decisions.[24] In high-stakes conversations, skilled physicians may need to partner with developmental experts (e.g., child life specialists) to support patients. Each person's expertise enhances SDM.[16] As the SDM process begins, explicitly stating that each participant will be open and forthcoming can set the stage for a discussion that addresses deeply held values and beliefs.

Time Constraints and Shared Decision Making

Clinicians are busy and SDM takes time. When available, decision aids can help physicians identify the appropriate information to share with families and to do so in a way that families find useful.[25] However, evidence-based decision aids do not exist for every decision. The broader a clinician's scope of practice is, the more challenging it will be to provide comprehensive and up-to-date information.

Conversations do not need to happen in one sitting. Raising the issue of a decision and eliciting values can occur at one time point, while the specifics of the options (and how they conflict or are compatible with a family's goals) can happen at another time.

System-Level Supports to Foster Shared Decision Making in Clinical Practice

System-level supports can be helpful in overcoming time constraints. One approach is to build SDM into clinic workflows. Systems have been set up using patient portals and/or email messaging and surveys to gather families' preferences and goals along with children's symptoms on a regular basis. Such approaches remove the burden of collecting this information from the clinical encounter. In a trial in persistent pediatric asthma, parents reported that a system that checked in monthly with them at home improved communication with the office and resulted in fewer parent-reported asthma flares for children and days of missed work for parents.[26,27] Similarly, in attention-deficit/hyperactivity disorder (ADHD), the implementation of an electronic system to gather preferences, goals, and symptoms fostered communication with teachers in schools.[28] One tertiary care pediatric hospital developed an institutional program to systematically support SDM.[29] The program made decision aids available to the public, taught clinicians to use decision-support strategies in practice, and offered independent decision-support services to patients and families. The program was supported by both parents and clinicians and led to improved satisfaction.[29]

Theory Contributions
to Building a Pragmatic Strategy for Shared
Decision Making

Although many conceptual models have been developed for SDM, multiple overlapping elements contribute to its pragmatic approach.[30] We will focus on the theoretical contributions related to the importance of building a trusting relationship between clinicians and patients, the recognition of patients and families as experts in their values, and the importance of building capacities for autonomous decision making in pediatric patients.

Building a Trusting Relationship Between Physicians and Families

Cultivating a trusting relationship between the individuals involved in SDM is central to its operationalization. We argue that one central goal of SDM is to create or further develop a trusting relationship between clinicians and patients and families that allows for the open sharing of information, values, and (if desired) recommendations from the physician. Physicians can engender trust by explicitly acknowledging their willingness to partner with their patients and through explicit statements of empathy.[31] In successful SDM, physicians must strive to be perceived as supportive of patients and families by listening and creating space for the families' values to drive the best plan for the patient.[32,33]

Patients and Families as Experts in Their Values

If equipoise exists, then recognition that the patient and family are experts in their values becomes essential. The clinician's role is to provide medical expertise and to contextualize the medical evidence in light of what is most important to the family. It is not possible for the physician to determine what is most important to a family without engaging them in a conversation about their values. While families may not be able to answer questions about their goals of care, they often are able to describe what they are hoping for, what they are worried about, and what it means to be a good parent to their child in this circumstance. It is the physician's responsibility to present the medical evidence in the context of these values as decision making proceeds.

Shared Decision Making and Relational Autonomy

Finally, an important aspect of SDM is to promote capacities for autonomy. The capacities for autonomy require cultivation and support by others in one's environment. Walter and Ross have articulated a set of capacities that make up a relational understanding of autonomy.[34] In this model, these capacities all depend upon others for their development and ongoing maintenance.

The ability to make decisions for oneself at any given time can only exist if previous decisions have been offered to the individual and the context around those decisions has been to some degree in the individual's control. If an individual makes a choice but others around them dismiss or override that choice consistently, then the ability to have confidence in their decision making will be hindered.

Another important aspect of relational autonomy is the perception of self-respect, which is intimately tied to others treating one respectfully. If a person is never given the respect of participating in decisions or having their values incorporated into decision making, they may not value or respect the importance of their own worth and role in decision making. People must learn this over a lifetime. Incorporating the child's perspective in decision making does not start in adolescence, but should be started as early as school age with explanations for why choices are being made and why these choices align with goals the parents and child have for the child.[35] Such an approach will allow an adolescent or an adult to participate in the process of SDM.

A Case Example for Shared Decision Making in an Adolescent

Jordan is a 15-year-old girl with a history of acute myeloid leukemia (AML) diagnosed 6 months previously. Because her leukemia was high risk, she had a bone marrow transplant as part of her treatment 2 months ago. She has received most of her treatments during multiple hospitalizations. She was in the intensive care unit (ICU) a few months ago when she had sepsis, an infection in her blood.

Three days ago, Jordan developed a fever at home and presented to the emergency department. She received antibiotics and medication to increase her blood pressure and she was admitted to the ICU. In the ICU, her breathing got worse and the ICU staff put a breathing tube in her airway and hooked her up to a ventilator. The blood counts drawn on admission showed "suspicious cells" that everyone worried could be leukemia cells. A repeat bone marrow test was done today that confirms an early relapse of her leukemia. Jordan had recovered to the point of being extubated so she can communicate, but her condition overall is still very tenuous. The oncologists do not believe they have any more standard cancer-directed therapies that would put her into remission, but they could determine her eligibility for clinical trials with other investigational therapies. Given the clinicians' equipoise about which path forward is appropriate, they want to discuss the options about next steps with Jordan and her parents.

Pragmatic Steps in Shared Decision Making

Drawing upon the barriers to SDM identified in the literature and some of the central aspects of the process described in its theoretical foundation, we have identified 10 distinct steps that we will outline to provide clear and specific recommendations for how to proceed in an SDM conversation.

1. Ask

In many circumstances, before having a discussion about which treatment plan to choose, new medical information must be conveyed to set the stage for the discussion. Because the information shared has a high probability of changing the patient's and family's understanding of their health and even identity, it should be approached as a giving-serious-news conversation. The first "ask" should be determining if all the people that need to hear the information are available and to what extent the parents want their child to be part of the initial conversation. For younger children, many parents request to hear the information first and then to have support in sharing the summary with their child. Asking Jordan's parents if it would be best to share the information with the whole family at the same time should be determined before moving forward.

The second part of the "ask" is assessing the patient's and family's current understanding of their health status. Asking simple questions like "What have the other doctors and nurses told you about your condition?" can be helpful in assessing what information has been previously absorbed as well as someone's level of health literacy. Many physicians trust that news has been shared with a family previously and start directly in with the new information. Without ascertaining a patient's understanding, there is a missed opportunity to address previously developed misconceptions or concerns that are central to a patient's perspective.

In addition to assessing the patient's or family's understanding of their health condition, it is also helpful to assess what kind of information they find most helpful—for example, "Some families prefer numbers and statistics, while other families want more of a big picture. What is most useful to you in learning new information?" When offering these options to families, it is important to explain that there is no one kind of information that is more appropriate, and that if other forms of information are desired later, the topic can be rediscussed using other kinds of information.

2. Tell (and Respond to Resulting Emotion)

After assessing a family's health literacy level, what they already understand about their health, and what kind of information is most helpful to them, physicians can then provide the new information relevant to an SDM conversation. Resources for communicating complicated concepts like risk and statistical probabilities and assessing understanding are available on the Agency for Healthcare and Research Quality's (AHRQ) SHARE website.[36] Best practice in providing serious news is to use a single concise sentence utilizing no jargon. In Jordan's case, the information can be as simple as "I wish I had different news, but the cancer is back and we have no more treatments that can cure it." Once the information has been conveyed, it is essential that the physician pause to allow for the expected emotional response from the patient and family. The emotion confirms that the physician has been adequately clear in conveying the main message. Emotion can manifest in a variety of ways including anger, crying, an anxious expression of multiple questions, and even completely shutting down with no engagement. Anticipating and then acknowledging emotion in any form is important. Explicit statements of empathy can help build the trusting relationship needed to proceed with the discussion, as well as help move the family from a highly emotional state to one where they can engage in further discussion. Useful expressions of empathy include naming the observed emotion ("This is overwhelming") and normalizing the experience for a patient or family ("Anyone hearing this news would be upset"). Another useful expression of empathy demonstrates the physician's respect for what the patient and family have been through: "It is clear you have had to deal with so much and you have supported each other through many difficult times already." Clinicians can also acknowledge how they will support the patient and family through this difficult process: "We will be with you on this journey and you are not alone in figuring out what to do next."

3. Second Ask

Before the conversation proceeds, it is important to look for cues from the family that they are ready to move forward and re-engage. Often, these signs are nonverbal, including more consistent eye contact. Sometimes the family asks an explicit question regarding what to do next. It is important to assess other pieces of information at this point. The second ask, "What questions do you have?," determines what information the patient and family have absorbed. If there are no questions, then physicians can try to determine what has been understood by asking the family, "I know we've already covered a lot of information. What will you share with other friends and family when they ask you what you heard?" This approach is less confrontational than a simple request of "What did I just tell you?" and can be framed as a support if the family worries about how they will share the news with others.

If the clinician is confident that the patient and family have understood the most important aspects of the new information, then it is possible to ask permission to discuss what the options are moving forward. Asking permission in this circumstance gives some control back to the family and might lead to a natural breaking point in the conversation if the family needs more time to process all that has already been shared or the visit needs to conclude due to other constraints.

4. More Than One Acceptable Option

Patients and families who have heard life-changing news may not realize that there is more than one option available to them moving forward. For families who have been receiving cancer-directed therapies, it may seem that the only path forward would be to pursue further cancer treatments. Clinicians must assess their own biases about whether they are in a position of equipoise and accept that different families may make different choices when hearing the full information about the options. If that is the case, then clinicians need to explain to patients and families that they are in a new situation, which allows for more than one loving path forward. Depending on what is most important to the family, they may choose one path over another.

5. Describe the Different Paths

For families to make an informed decision, the clinician needs to offer a clear description of the paths forward. It is important to provide the medical facts without too much value judgment of which option is the preferred one from the clinician's perspective. It can be helpful to start the discussion with, "Loving families make different choices depending on what is most important to them. I will support you in whichever path you choose." In Jordan's case, this may include one path of continued cancer-directed therapies including investigational agents that could extend the length of life but cause side effects and more time in the hospital. An alternative path would be a shift toward a comfort-focused approach that would allow for more time at home with symptom-focused care that may improve the quality of life while shortening the length. Additionally, using a best-case, worst-case, and most-likely-case scenario can be helpful in providing a clear vision for what each path may look like.[37] If the best-case scenario in one path is worse than a family can imagine, then it is probably not the right path for them.

6. Elicit Concerns or Questions

The information provided about the different paths can be overwhelming and retrigger an emotional response. Clinicians should carefully track the emotional responses to make sure the family is able to absorb the data that is conveyed. Eliciting questions and concerns about the different paths can allow reassessment of understanding and clarify anything that was not clearly conveyed. An example is, "Can you tell me what you understand a comfort-focused approach to be at this point?"

7. Elicit Values

It is essential to SDM that clinicians work to elicit patient and family values in light of the different clinical options that have been presented. While many families may not know how to respond to a question like "What are your goals for your child's care?," they often can articulate things that they are hoping for or worried about. It can be useful to ask these questions explicitly and then track the concerns, later asking clarifying questions about what concerns them most. Another helpful set of questions can be, "What does it mean to be a good parent to your child now in light of this new information?" and "What would you regret the most if it didn't happen?" Reflecting back to families what has been heard is a good way for the clinician to track and validate their concerns. Particularly for concerns raised, it can be helpful to acknowledge that "Many parents I talk to in these circumstances are worried about this." If families are unable to articulate concerns, this phrase can also be helpful in giving words to some of the negative emotions that people may have difficulty saying out loud. Giving permission and normalizing these worries can be helpful to articulating the full range of concerns and hopes a family has.

In circumstances where adolescents are part of the process, it is essential to elicit their values and concerns in addition to those of their parents. If parents are used to speaking for their child, it can be helpful to set the expectation that "We always want to ask the patient about what is important to them as well. We know this is happening to them and their body and they are the experts in what this experience is for them." Utilizing child life specialists and art therapists to help adolescents process serious news and be able to articulate their values is also essential, since they may have a harder time processing the long-term implications in situations of high emotion and are prone to experience significant anxiety.[38]

8. Determine How Much Pediatric Clinician Input Is Desired in Decision Making

Families and patients have different expectations for how much input they want from their clinicians in making decisions. In this process, families need to determine who wants to participate in the decision making and in what capacity. Some families want the physician to provide a recommendation for which path to choose, and others want the clinicians to merely provide information about the different options but will decide with the support of family and friends; it is important to assess whether the patient and family would like an explicit recommendation or not. The SDM process does not require physician recommendations, but a relational autonomy approach to decision making would support a recommendation from the clinician if the recommendation was based upon the values expressed by the patient and family.[39] Offering one when it is not requested could be seen as undue pressure to choose the option recommended. It is also possible that families may want to defer decision making entirely to the provider or that adolescent patients will defer the decision entirely to their parents. Delaying decision making is always an available option in SDM, though clinical circumstances, especially in the ICU setting, may limit options if decision making is delayed.

9. Make a Recommendation, if Appropriate, and Ask for a Decision

After determining who will participate in choosing a path forward, it is important to ask which path the patient or family prefers at this time. If the family would like a recommendation from the clinical team, it is appropriate at this time to offer it. The recommendation should be based on the values that have been articulated by the family. If values conflict between the patient and parents, it might be an important time to further discuss how the family makes decisions in these circumstances and whether the parents are hearing the child's concerns. These situations can be difficult to navigate, but a mediated approach for older adolescents to ensure that what is driving their disagreement is discussed more openly can lead to a unified plan for how to proceed in most circumstances, although outliers do exist. Ensuring adolescents and parents receive adequate psychologic supports in life-threatening circumstances like Jordan's is essential to navigating these complicated decisions.[24]

10. Plan for Follow-Up

To demonstrate ongoing support for patients and families, it is important to acknowledge either the decision that has been arrived at or that the conversations can be continued at another time with a decision delayed until then, if clinically possible. For decisions around changes in the direction of treatment, it may be necessary to involve subspecialty services, like palliative care, to provide more clear information about possible paths forward like hospice care. When a decision can be life altering, it is important to indicate that families can choose one path now, like cancer-directed therapy, but can choose an alternative path in the future if the symptoms become too burdensome. Setting expectations about whether decisions will be revisited in the future can alleviate anxiety that it would be difficult to change course if needed, but also prepare parents that these challenging conversations may need to be rediscussed in light of clinical worsening.

Conclusion

Despite recommendations by the National Academy of Sciences[1] and multiple professional organizations[2] to implement SDM strategies, use remains low. Though system-level supports and institutional initiatives can support SDM implementation and facilitate the inclusion of the patient and family perspective in decision making, clinician knowledge and comfort with SDM must continue to increase to promote broader use of SDM. With an example from pediatric oncology and intensive care, this chapter highlights a pragmatic approach to realize SDM in practice through a series of key communication behaviors. Consistent clinician implementation of these approaches that can be generalized to varied settings would represent an important advance in realizing SDM in pediatric care.

References

1. Institute of Medicine. *Crossing the Quality Chasm: A New Health System for the 21st Century*. National Academies Press; 2001.
2. Adams RC, Levy SE. Shared decision-making and children with disabilities: pathways to consensus. *Pediatrics.* 2017 Jun;139(6):e20170956.
3. Fiks A, Mayne S, Localio R, Alessandrini E, Guevara J. Shared decision-making and health care expenditures among children with special health care needs. *Pediatrics.* 2012;129:99.
4. Sleath B, Carpenter D, Syner R, et al. Child and caregiver involvement and shared decision-making during asthma pediatric visits. *J Asthma.* 2011;48(10):1022–1031.
5. Legare F, Ratte S, Gravel K, Graham ID. Barriers and facilitators to implementing shared decision-making in clinical practice: update of a systematic review of health professionals' perceptions. *Patient Educ Couns.* 2008;73(3):526–535.
6. Wyatt KD, List B, Brinkman WB, et al. Shared decision making in pediatrics: a systematic review and meta-analysis. *Acad Pediatr.* 2015;15(6):573–583.
7. Legare F, Ratte S, Stacey D, et al. Interventions for improving the adoption of shared decision making by healthcare professionals. *Cochrane Database Syst Rev.* 2010;5:CD006732.
8. Legare F, Turcotte S, Stacey D, Ratte S, Kryworuchko J, Graham ID. Patients' perceptions of sharing in decision: a systematic review of interventions to enhance shared decision making in routine clinical practice. *Patient.* 2012;5(1):1–19.
9. Yin H, Dreyer B, Vivar K, MacFarland S, van Schaick L, Medndelsohn A. Perceived barriers to care and attitudes towards shared decision-making among low socioeconomic status parents: role of health literacy. *Acad Pediatr.* 2012;12(2):117–124.
10. Cabana M, Rand C, Powe N, Wu A, Wilson M, Abbound F. Why don't physicians follow clinical practice guidelines? A framework for improvement. *JAMA.* 1999;282:1458–1465.
11. Fiks A. Contrasting parents' and pediatricians' perspectives on shared decision-making in ADHD. *Pediatrics.* 2010;127:e88.
12. Hudak P, Frankel R, Braddock C, Nisenbaum R, Luca P, McKeever C. Do patients' communication behaviors provide insight into their preferences for participation in decision making? *Med Decis Making.* 2008;28:385–393.
13. Bruera E, Willey J, Palmer JL, Rosales M. Treatment decisions for breast carcinoma: patient preferences and physician perceptions. *Cancer.* 2002;94:2076–2080.

14. Fiks AG, Hughes C, Gafen A, Guevara JP, Barg F. Contrasting parents' and pediatricians' perspectives on shared decision making in ADHD. *Pediatrics*. 2011;127:e188–e196.

15. Smith SK, Dixon A, Trevena L, Nutbeam D, McCaffery KJ. Exploring patient involvement in healthcare decision making across different education and functional health literacy groups. *Soc Sci Med*. 2009;69(12):1805–1812.

16. Boland L, Graham ID, Legare F, et al. Barriers and facilitators of pediatric shared decision-making: a systematic review. *Implement Sci*. 2019;14(7):1–25.

17. Frosch DL, May SG, Rendle KA, Tietbohl C, Elwyn G. Authoritarian physicians and patients' fear of being labeled 'difficult' among key obstacles to shared decision making. *Health Aff*. 2012;31(5):1030–1038.

18. Makoul G, Clayman ML. An integrative model of shared decision making in medical encounters. *Patient Educ Couns*. 2006;60(3):301–303.

19. Elwyn G, Frosch D, Thomson R, et al. Shared decision making: a model for clinical practice. *J Gen Intern Med*. 2012;27(10):1361–1367.

20. Back AL, Arnold RM, Baile WF, et al. Efficacy of communication skills training for giving bad news and discussing transitions to palliative care. *Arch Intern Med*. 2007;167(5):453.

21. Parker RM, Ratzan SC, Lurie N. Health literacy: a policy challenge for advancing high-quality health care. *Health Aff (Millwood)*. 2003;22(4):147–153.

22. Institute of Medicine Committee on Health Literacy. In Nielsen-Bohlman L, Panzer AM, Kindig DA (Eds). *Health Literacy: A Prescription to End Confusion*. Washington, DC: National Academies Press; 2004.

23. Walter JK, Faerber J, Odeniyi F, et al. *Health Literacy and Pediatric Shared Decision-Making Preferences and Styles*. Paper presented at Pediatric Academic Society, Vancouver, BC, Canada, 2014.

24. Halpern J. Creating the safety and respect necessary for "shared" decision-making. *Pediatrics*. 2018;142(Suppl 3):S163–S169.

25. Brinkman W, Majcher J, Poling L, et al. Shared decision-making to improve attention-deficit hyperactivity disorder care. *Patient Educ Couns*. 2013;93(1):95–101.

26. Fiks AG, Mayne SL, Karavite DJ, et al. Parent-reported outcomes of a shared decision-making portal in asthma: a practice-based RCT. *Pediatrics*. 2015;135(4):e965–e973.

27. Fiks AG, Mayne S, Karavite DJ, DeBartolo E, Grundmeier RW. A shared e-decision support portal for pediatric asthma. *J Ambul Care Manage*. 2014;37(2):120–126.

28. Fiks AG, Mayne SL, Michel JJ, et al. Distance-learning, ADHD quality improvement in primary care: a cluster-randomized trial. *J Dev Behav Pediatr*. 2017;38(8):573–583.

29. Boland L, McIsaac DI, Lawson ML. Barriers to and facilitators of implementing shared decision making and decision support in a paediatric hospital: a descriptive study. *Paediatr Child Health.* 2016;21(3):e17–e21.

30. Legare F, Adekpedjou R, Stacey D, et al. Interventions for increasing the use of shared decision making by healthcare professionals. *Cochrane Database Syst Rev.* 2018;7:CD006732.

31. Madrigal VN, Kelly KP. Supporting family decision-making for a child who is seriously ill: creating synchrony and connection. *Pediatrics.* 2018;142(Suppl 3):S170–S177.

32. Elwyn G, Edwards A, Kinnersley P, Grol R. Shared decision making and the concept of equipoise: the competences of involving patients in health-care choices. *Br J Gen Pract.* 2000;50(460):892–899.

33. Stiggelbout AM, Van der Weijden T, De Wit MP, et al. Shared decision making: really putting patients at the centre of healthcare. *BMJ (Online).* 2012;344.

34. Walter JK, Ross LF. Relational autonomy as the key to effective behavioral change. *Philos Psychiatr Psychol.* 2013;20(2):169–177.

35. Committee on Bioethics. Informed consent in decision-making in pediatric practice. *Pediatrics.* 2016;138(2).

36. Agency for Healthcare Research and Quality (AHRQ). The SHARE Approach. https://www.ahrq.gov/professionals/education/curriculum-tools/shareddecisionmaking/index.html. Published 2017. Updated February 2017. Accessed August 15, 2017.

37. Taylor LJ, Nabozny MJ, Steffens NM, et al. A framework to improve surgeon communication in high-stakes surgical decisions: best case/worst case. *JAMA Surg.* 2017;152(6):531–538.

38. Diekema D. Adolescent refusal of lifesaving treatment: are we asking the right questions? *Adolesc Med.* 2011;22:213–228.

39. Walter JK, Ross LF. Relational autonomy: moving beyond limits of isolated individualism. *Pediatrics.* 2014;133:S16–S23.

8

The Role of Children and Adolescents in Decision Making About Life-Threatening Illness

Victoria A. Miller and Melissa K. Cousino

The concept of shared decision making (SDM) was developed in relation to the adult patient-provider relationship and entails mutuality, reciprocal information giving and decision making, and agreement about the decision.[1] These characteristics do not necessarily apply to the child-provider relationship in pediatric settings. When a child is the patient, parents are typically the primary decision maker, because they are legally responsible for health care decision making, and children's communication and decision-making abilities are still developing. As a result, children may not be equal partners in decision making and may not be willing or able to share opinions, preferences, and values; disclose clinically relevant information; and evaluate options. These behaviors are necessary according to a widely cited model of SDM.[1]

The concept of decision-making involvement (DMI) is more appropriate than SDM when referring to child and adolescent patients, because it assumes that children still need to learn about and practice decision making.[2,3] DMI refers to the multiple ways that children can be engaged in decisions, which may include active participation of the child (e.g., asking for advice, expressing opinions or concerns), adult provision of information, and adult solicitation of the child's preferences, questions, or concerns.[4] This definition, which underscores the relational aspects of decision making,[5] recognizes that collaborative decision making plays an important role in normative development. It also appreciates the role of adults in supporting children's involvement in the decision-making process and facilitating independent and effective decision making as they mature. The concept of DMI reflects that parents and health care providers offer support and guidance to children, even as children become increasingly independent with respect to making decisions.[6] This developmental approach is critical, as prior research suggests that while youth want to be involved in treatment decision making,[7] they also desire adult input[8] and feel that decision-making independence, without support or guidance, can be burdensome.[9]

The concept of DMI also differs from SDM because it recognizes that children and adolescents need exposure to and practice with decision making before they will be able to make decisions on their own. Involvement in decision making may enable children to learn about the pros and cons of different options, the potential outcomes of alternatives, and the communication skills needed to share in decision making. Furthermore, DMI may facilitate self-efficacy,[10] promote cooperation with treatment, and enhance coping.[11,12] Adolescents are more satisfied after visits to the doctor when the doctor has a patient-centered style of decision making.[13] They are also more adherent with doctor recommendations.[14] Given the loss of control children and adolescents typically feel when diagnosed with a serious, life-threatening illness, DMI may be especially important.[15] Furthermore, children have reported that they feel more valued when involved in discussions with health care providers.[16] Prior research assessing DMI in the context of parent-child interactions about chronic illness management decisions found that when youth with type 1 diabetes were more involved by expressing opinions, sharing illness-related information, and negotiating or brainstorming with parents, they had better treatment adherence, after controlling for age.[17] In a longitudinal study with youth with type 1 diabetes, aspects of DMI were associated with adherence and interacted with age to predict glycemic control.[18] Given that nonadherence rates in pediatric chronic illness are high and can have serious short- and long-term consequences,[19,20] facilitating youth's involvement in illness-related decisions may be an important target for interventions to improve adherence and health outcomes. Involving youth may also lay the groundwork for increased responsibility and successful transition to adult health care.[21]

Focusing on DMI instead of SDM is consistent with the American Academy of Pediatrics (AAP) policy related to informed consent, parental permission, and assent and Clinical Report on SDM with children with disabilities and their caregivers. [22] These documents state that the experiences and perspectives of children are critical; thus, children should be involved to the extent that they are able to enhance outcomes, such as increased trust and improved health. Furthermore, the AAP 2016 policy suggests that providers should not expect children's and adolescents' decision making to be autonomous or voluntary, because parental influence is developmentally appropriate.

Potential Challenges to Involving Children

Decision making about serious illness occurs against the dynamic backdrop of developmental change, as well as individual and family differences, such as prior experience with decision making, health-related goals, coping style, cultural background, family structure, and parenting style.[23] Developmental factors have been discussed at length elsewhere.[24,25] and include cognitive development (e.g., attention, memory, abstract thinking, and reasoning), psychosocial maturity (e.g., future orientation and impulsivity), and decision-making and communication skills. Furthermore, children may desire more or less information and DMI with changes in maturity, experience, and health status. Involving children may also vary based on characteristics of the decision to be made, such as urgency, risk/benefit ratio, certainty of the outcome, number of options available, setting in which the decision is being made, and the extent to which the decision is preference sensitive.

In addition to the shifting landscape of development and variability in decisions, there are several additional barriers to DMI, such as lack of time,[26] a history of parents as the primary focus of communication,[27] and parental interference.[28] In the majority of cases, parents are in an ideal position to facilitate communication between children and providers, because they understand the broader context of the child or adolescent's preferences, values, and goals; can provide emotional support through the process of decision making; and are highly involved in implementing decisions. However, balancing the needs and preferences of both parents and children may be difficult, especially if they are discordant. Parents typically serve as gatekeepers of information and may constrain provider communication with children about treatment decisions by limiting what the child can be told, due to their desire to shield the child from distressing information and promote a hopeful outlook.[29] In addition to constraining children's involvement, the desire to protect the child from distress may impact parental understanding or willingness to ask questions when prognostic information and treatment decisions are discussed with providers. The tendency to limit the child's DMI may be strong at the time of diagnosis of a life-threatening illness. It may shift to more partnership with the child over the course of the illness.[30]

Facilitating Child and Adolescent Decision-Making Involvement

Involving Children During Office Visits and Hospitalizations

Patient-provider communication provides the foundation for decision making by enabling sharing of information, discussion of options, and exchange of opinions and preferences. There are several potential communication strategies for involving children and adolescents in decision making, including turn-taking (e.g., teaching and encouraging the child to take turns speaking,[31]) asking the child for relevant information (e.g., symptoms, barriers to adherence), providing information directly to the child while avoiding medical jargon, soliciting questions, inviting the child's opinion regarding aspects of treatment, and checking for understanding (Box 8.1). Prior studies have found that when providers use these communication strategies, children verbally participate more during the encounter.[32] It is important to let children know when a decision is not theirs to make, but providers and parents should offer other choices that are related to treatment. For example, while children may not have a choice about starting chemotherapy for newly diagnosed leukemia, they can make the decision about how to manage hair loss.[33]

Providers should explore their own beliefs about how children should or should not be involved in decision making, because these beliefs will shape their behavior when communicating with youth. For example, providers may think that youth are unable to make certain decisions about life-threatening illness[34] or expect that youth do not want to be involved, which may limit their attempts to communicate directly with youth and engage them in decision making. It would be helpful to assess children's preferences by asking them how they wish to be involved and what kinds of information they want and to reassess these preferences over time. Some

---

Box 8.1 Strategies for Involving Children and Adolescents in Decision Making

---

Communication Behaviors
- Assess preferences for information and involvement
- Teach turn-taking
- Ask for information directly from child
- Provide information directly to child
- Solicit questions
- Ask for child's opinion or concerns
- Assess understanding
- Avoid offering a choice if that choice cannot or will not be honored
- Offer "smaller" choices related to decision
- Be attuned to emotional responses to information
- Reassess preferences with changes in development, experience, and health status
- Provide guidance to parents for involving children in health-related decision making

Tools for Facilitating Discussions About End-of-Life Care
- *My CHATT* (Cousino, Rea, & Mednick, 2017)
- *My Wishes* (Aging with Dignity, 2015)
- *This Is My World* (Zadeh & Wiener, 2011)

---

youth may not respond to attempts to involve them in discussions or decisions (e.g., the inhibited 7-year-old who wants parents to answer for him). Such lack of engagement may reflect a desire to avoid emotionally distressing information or reduce anxiety and should be respected. At the same time, efforts to engage youth should not be entirely abandoned, because youth's preferences will change with development, with different types of decisions, and over the course of the illness. Furthermore, when providers make efforts to involve children, it conveys that the child has a role to play and may enhance the child's comfort speaking up during future interactions.[35]

Providers can also support youth and families in illness-related decision making that occurs outside of the medical setting, such as when and how to balance treatments with the demands of daily life, responding to symptoms (e.g., identifying and responding to low blood sugar in youth with type 1 diabetes), managing pain, determining activities based on symptoms or potential health consequences, and deciding whether and how to discuss the illness with others. Providers can explain to parents that involving youth in decision-making discussions can be beneficial and coach them to ask for the child's opinion, provide information, solicit questions, and maintain balance between the child's responsibility for managing treatments and parental supervision. Guidance from providers about appropriate child responsibility is important, because adherence may decline when youth have independence for managing treatments before they are developmentally ready.[36] Providers can directly support youth by helping them to distinguish between decisions and tasks they can manage independently and those for which they should seek guidance from a parent or other adult and to plan ahead for high-risk situations that may negatively impact health or treatment adherence (e.g., situations involving peer pressure or emotional arousal).

Involving Children and Adolescents in End-of-Life Decision Making

The 2014 Institute of Medicine (IOM) report "Dying in America: Improving Quality and Honoring Individual Preferences Near End of Life" highlighted a critical need to improve the DMI of seriously ill children and adolescents in advance care planning and end-of-life decision making.[37] Emerging literature suggests that many young people with chronic illness prefer to be involved in decision making about their end-of-life care if seriously ill.[38] For example, among adolescents with cancer and heart failure, 75% and 83%, respectively, indicated a preference to be involved in their end-of-life decision making.[39] In addition to reporting a preference for end-of-life DMI, pilot studies suggest that young people are often capable of understanding complex end-of-life decision making (e.g., adoption of a do-not-resuscitate order, transition to comfort care), as well as the consequences of such decisions (e.g., impact of decision on their loved ones.)[40] In a novel randomized controlled trial of a family-centered advance care planning intervention for adolescents and young adults with cancer, the majority of participants (91%) found their structured involvement in advance care planning to be helpful.[41] Furthermore, youth DMI of this nature may contribute to reductions in invasive interventions at a child's end of life, increased home-based deaths, and reduced decisional burden among family members.[42]

Despite a preference for end-of-life DMI among a majority of children and adolescents, patients, providers, and parents report that conversations with youth about end-of-life decision making occur at much lower rates.[43] Many barriers exist to discussing end-of-life decision making, such as provider discomfort, concerns about decreasing hope, and parental preferences to withhold such information and/or DMI.

In addition to the strategies described previously, the literature outlines approaches for engaging young people in discussions about end-of-life decision making. Rosenberg and colleagues underscore the importance of cultural humility, timing, and content.[38] Prior to engaging youth in end-of-life DMI, one should first understand a young person's and their family's cultural and religious beliefs, if any. Assessing both patient and parent preferences for information giving and youth DMI in end-of-life care is a critical next step. A provider can simply start by asking, "How do you like to receive information about your health? Make decisions about your care?" The patient-reported *My CHATT* tool can also facilitate discussion about communication and decision-making preferences specific to end-of-life care.[44] Providers should establish consistent time points for when preferences for end-of-life DMI are assessed and revisited (e.g., diagnosis, reoccurrence or progression of disease). Given the challenges of prognostication in pediatric critical illness, honest and systematic conversations that occur throughout the disease trajectory decrease unexpected decision-making discussions during highly stressful times.[45] Thus, it can be helpful to say to patients and their families, "I want to be sure that we discuss things and involve you in decisions that are important to you. This may even include talking about difficult topics sometimes, like what you would want if you could not speak for yourself. Every now and then, I will check in to see if your preferences for discussing these things have changed."

After obtaining background information about the child's and family's preferences, beliefs, values, and disease knowledge, the communication to follow about end-of-life DMI should be direct, compassionate, honest, and developmentally appropriate.[38] Leading researchers and clinicians in the fields of pediatric oncology and palliative care have outlined various phrases for discussing end-of-life decision making with children and their families that serve as helpful resources.[46,47] In addition, a handful of clinical tools exist for facilitating such conversations, such as *This Is My World*,[48] and *My CHATT*.[44]

It is important to highlight that while the majority of young people with critical illnesses state a preference for end-of-life DMI, a subset may not desire such involvement. For example, 12% of teens with cancer stated they were uncomfortable/did not want to talk about death.[49] Similarly, 17% of teens with heart failure preferred that their parents make all end-of-life-related decisions.[39] Thus, one must always practice with keen awareness that each child and family is unique, and various factors, such as illness experiences, family beliefs, and developmental level, can change and influence one's end-of-life decision-making preferences over time.

Summary

The concept of DMI, which recognizes the developmental and relational context of child and adolescent decision making, is more appropriate than SDM in the context of pediatric decision making. By utilizing the concept of DMI instead of SDM, we avoid propagating both a lack of conceptual clarity in the literature and inattention to the developmental context of child/adolescent decision making in both research and clinical endeavors. DMI allows children to observe, learn, and practice making decisions, without bearing full responsibility for the decision to be made, and may enhance control, self-efficacy, and adherence. When providers attempt to involve youth in decision making, youth learn that their perspective matters, which may increase the likelihood that they will participate in the future. Providers can involve children and adolescents in multiple ways, and involvement should evolve based on development, preferences, type of decision, and health status. Despite its importance, youth involvement in communication and decision making in medical settings appears to be low. Additional research is needed to identify and understand reasons for children's low involvement and develop and evaluate provider-, parent-, and/ or youth-focused strategies to enhance different aspects of DMI in multiple settings and contexts as children develop.

References

1. Charles C, Gafni A, Whelan T. Shared decision-making in the medical encounter: what does it mean? (or it takes at least two to tango). *Soc Sci Med*. 1997;44(5):681–692.

2. Rogoff B. *Apprenticeship in Thinking*. New York: Oxford University Press; 1990.

3. Ruhe KM, De Clercq E, Wangmo T, Elger BS. Relational capacity: broadening the notion of decision-making capacity in paediatric healthcare. *Bioethical Inq*. 2016;13(4):515–524.

4. Miller VA, Harris D. Measuring children's decision making involvement regarding chronic illness management. *J Pediatr Psychol*. 2012;37(3):292–306.

5. Miller VA, Reynolds WW, Nelson RM. Parent-child roles in decision-making about medical research. *Ethics Behav.18*, 2008;(2–3):161–181.

6. Fuligni AJ, Eccles JS. Perceived parent-child relationships and early adolescents' orientation toward peers. *Dev Psychol*. 1993;29(4):622–632.

7. Knopf JM, Hornung RW, Slap GB, DeVellis RF, Britto MT. Views of treatment decision making from adolescents with chronic illnesses and their parents: a pilot study. *Health Expect*. 2008;11(4):343–354.

8. Lipstein EA, Muething KA, Dodds CM, Britto MT. "I'm the one taking it": adolescent participation in chronic disease treatment decisions. *J Adolesc Health*. 2013;53(2):253–259.

9. Miller VA. Parent-child collaborative decision making for the management of chronic illness: a qualitative analysis. *Fam Syst Health*. 2009;27(3):249–266.

10. White F. Parent-adolescent communication and adolescent decision-making. *J Fam Stud*. 1996;2(1):41–56.

11. Drotar D, Crawford P, Bonner M. Collaborative decision-making and promoting treatment adherence in pediatric chronic illness. *Patient Intell*. 2010;2:1–7.

12. Schmidt S, Petersen C, Bullinger M. Coping with chronic disease from the perspective of children and adolescents-a conceptual framework and its implications for participation. *Child: Care Health Dev*. 2003;29(1):63–75.

13. Freed LH, Ellen JM, Irwin CE, Millstein SG. Determinants of adolescents' satisfaction with health care providers and intentions to keep follow-up appointments. *J Adolesc Health*. 1998;22(6):475–479.

14. Kyngas H, Rissanen M. Support as a crucial predictor of good compliance of adolescents with a chronic disease. *J Clin Nurs*. 2001;10(6):767–774.

15. Kelly KP, Mowbray C, Pyke-Grimm K, Hinds PS. Identifying a conceptual shift in child and adolescent-reported treatment decision making: "having a say, as I need it at this time." *Pediatr Blood Cancer*. 2017;64:e26262.

16. Angst DB, Deatrick JA. Involvement in health care decisions: parents and children with chronic illness. *J Fam Nurs*. 1996;2(2):174–194.

17. Miller VA, Jawad A. Relationship of youth involvement in diabetes-related decisions to treatment adherence. *J Clin Psychol Med Settings.* 2014;21(2):183–189.
18. Miller VA, Jawad AJ. Decision making involvement and prediction of adherence in youth with type 1 diabetes: a cohort sequential study. *J Pediatr Psychol.* 2019;44(1):61–71.
19. Bender B, Milgrom H, Rand C, Ackerson L. Psychological factors associated with medication nonadherence in asthmatic children. *J Asthma.* 1998;35(4):347–353.
20. Kovacs M, Obrosky DS, Goldston D, Drash A. Major depressive disorder in youths with IDDM: a controlled prospective study of course and outcome. *Diabetes Care.* 1997;20(1):45–51.
21. Monaghan M, Hilliard M, Sweenie R, Riekert K. Transition readiness in adolescents and emerging adults with diabetes: the role of patient-provider communication. *Curr Diab Rep.* 2013;13(6):900–908.
22. Adams RC, Levy SE, Council on Children with Disabilities. Shared decision-making and children with disabilities: pathways to consensus. *Pediatrics.* 2017;139(6):1–9.
23. Broome ME, Richards DJ. The influence of relationships on children's and adolescents' participation in research. *Nurs Res.* 2003;52(3):191–197.
24. Grootens-Wiegers P, Hein IM, van den Broek JM, De Vries MC. Medical decision-making in children and adolescents: developmental and neuroscientific aspects. *BMC Pediatr.* 2017;17(1):120.
25. McCabe MA. Involving children and adolescents in medical decision making: developmental and clinical considerations. *J Pediatr Psychol.* 1996;21(4):505–516.
26. Coyne I. Children's participation in consultations and decision-making at health service level: a review of the literature. *Int J Nurs Stud.* 2008;45(11):1682–1689.
27. van Staa A, On Your Own Feet Research Group. Unraveling triadic communication in hospital consultations with adolescents with chronic conditions: the added value of mixed methods research. *Patient Educ Couns.* 2011;82(3):455–464.
28. Beresford BA, Sloper P. Chronically ill adolescents' experiences of communicating with doctors: a qualitative study. *J Adolesc Health.* 2003;33(3):172–179.
29. Wangmo T, De Clercq E, Ruhe KM, et al. Better to know than to imagine: including children in their health care. *AJOB Empir Bioeth.* 2017;8(1):11–20.

30. Young B, Dixon-Woods M, Windridge KC, Heney D. Managing communication with young people who have a potentially life threatening chronic illness: qualitative study of patients and parents. *BMJ*. 2003;326:305–309.

31. Butz AM, Walker JM, Pulsifer M, Winkelstein M. Shared decision making in school-age children with asthma. *Pediatr Nurs*. 2007;33(2):111–116.

32. Miller VA, Werner-Lin A, Walser SA, Biswas S, Bernhardt B. An observational study of children's involvement in informed consent for exome sequencing research. *J Empir Res Hum Res Ethics*. 2017;12(1):6–13.

33. Coyne I, Amory A, Kiernan G, Gibson F. Children's participation in shared decision-making: children, adolescents, parents and healthcare professionals' perspectives and experiences. *Eur J Oncol Nurs*. 2014;18:273–280.

34. de Vries MC, Wit JM, Engberts DP, Kaspers GJL, van Leeuwen E. Pediatric oncologists' attitudes towards involving adolescents in decision-making concerning research participation. *Pediatr Blood Cancer*. 2010;55:123–128.

35. Edwards A, Elwyn G. Inside the black box of shared decision making: distinguishing between the process of involvement and who makes the decision. *Health Expect*. 2006;9(4):307–320.

36. Silva K, Miller VA. The role of cognitive and psychosocial maturity in type 1 diabetes management. *J Adolesc Health*. 2019. doi.org/10.1016/j.jadohealth.2018.10.294

37. Institute of Medicine. *Dying in America: Improving Quality and Honoring Individual Preferences Near the End of Life*. National Academies Press, Washington, DC. 2014.

38. Rosenberg AR, Wolfe J, Wiener L, Lyon M, Feudtner C. Ethics, emotions, and the skills of talking about progressing disease with terminally ill adolescents a review. *JAMA Pediatr*. 2016. https://doi.org/10.1001/jamapediatrics.2016.2142

39. Cousino MK, Miller VA, Smith C, et al. Medical and end-of-life decision making in adolescents' pre-heart transplant: a descriptive pilot study. *Palliat Med*. 2020 Mar;34(3):272–280.

40. Hinds PS, Drew D, Oakes LL, et al. End-of-life care preferences of pediatric patients with cancer. *J Clin Oncol*. 2005;23(36):9146–9154. https://doi.org/10.1200/JCO.2005.10.538

41. Lyon ME, Jacobs S, Briggs L, Cheng Y, Wang J. Family-centered advance care planning for teens with cancer. *JAMA Pediatr*. 2013;167(5):460–467. http://dx.doi.org/10.1001/jamapediatrics.2013.943

42. Lotz JD, Jox RJ, Borasio GD, Fuhrer M. Pediatric advance care planning: a systematic review. *Pediatrics*. 2013;131(3):e873–e880. https://doi.org/10.1542/peds.2012-2394

43. Cousino MK, Schumacher KR, Magee JC, et al. Communication about prognosis and end-of-life in pediatric organ failure and transplantation. *Pediatr Transplant*. 2019 May;23(3):e13373.

44. Cousino MK, Rea KE, Mednick LM. Understanding the healthcare communication needs of pediatric patients through the My CHATT tool: a pilot study. *J Commun Healthc*. 2017;10(1):16–21. https://doi.org/10.1080/17538068.2017.1278637

45. Wiener L, Zadeh S, Wexler LH, Pao M. When silence is not golden: engaging adolescents and young adults in discussions around end-of-life care choices. *Pediatr Blood Cancer*. 2013;60(5):715–718.

46. Blazin L, Cecchini C, Habashy C, Kaye E, Baker J. Communicating effectively in pediatric cancer care: translating evidence into practice. *Children*. 2018;5(3):40.

47. Sisk BA, Bluebond-Langner M, Wiener L, Mack J, Wolfe J. Prognostic disclosures to children: a historical perspective. *Pediatrics*. 2016;138(3):e20161278. https://doi.org/10.1542/peds.2016-1278

48. Zadeh S, Wiener L. *This Is My World*. 2nd ed. Bethesda, MD: National Institutes of Mental Health; 2011.

49. Jacobs S, Perez J, Cheng YI, Sill A, Wang J, Lyon ME. Adolescent end of life preferences and congruence with their parents' preferences: results of a survey of adolescents with cancer. *Pediatr Blood Cancer*. 2015;62(4):710–714. https://doi.org/10.1002/pbc.25358

9

A Stepwise Framework for Shared Decision Making in Pediatrics

Kimberly E. Sawyer and Douglas J. Opel

Shared decision making (SDM) is a well-established component of patient-centered care[1] and has been defined as decision making in which "both parties share information[,] . . . take steps to build consensus about the preferred treatment, and [reach an agreement] on the treatment to implement."[2] SDM has origins in the patient rights movement[3] and the concept of self-determination[4–6] that have emerged as a result of medical, cultural, and societal shifts over the last several decades.[2] Tools that facilitate SDM have been shown to improve patient knowledge of options, outcomes, and risk as well as patient selection of the option that matches their values.[7] Consequently, SDM has the potential to empower patients, enhance transparency, increase trust,[8] and improve health outcomes.[9,10]

However, there remain multiple barriers to implementing SDM. First, there are measurement barriers. Though many SDM measurement tools exist, the quality of these tools is lacking.[11] This has made it difficult to assess the impact of SDM on behavioral and health outcomes, with mixed results reported by investigators conducting recent systematic reviews.[12,13] Second, conceptual barriers exist. For instance, where the balance lies in SDM between patient autonomy and physician duty to promote the patient's best interest is still being debated.[14–22] Finally, practical barriers exist. It remains unclear how to use SDM in complex situations involving longitudinal interventions, multiple decision makers, and preventive treatments and/or with public health dimensions.[23-27]

How SDM translates to pediatric settings is even less understood.[28] Current SDM models do not completely address the unique features of pediatric decision making, such as the essential role of someone other than the patient—a surrogate decision maker (i.e., the parent or legal guardian)—in SDM. The presence of surrogates in SDM can impact how "shared" a decision can be in pediatrics since the range of potential decisions made by a surrogate is constrained by physician obligations to ensure surrogate decision making promotes the patient's best interest. Such differences can cause confusion about when and how to apply SDM in pediatric practice.[29-31]

Framework

The objective of this chapter is to contribute to the conceptual work needed in SDM and describe a practical framework for applying SDM in pediatrics. This framework adapts prior conceptual work on SDM in the adult setting[21,22,25,32-39] using methods in medical ethics[40] to account for decisional and contextual differences in pediatric decision making, such as the role and authority of parents in decision making for nonadolescent children.[18,22,38,41-43] This chapter also reflects refinements to the original published framework.[44] We focused these refinements on (1) distinguishing the concepts of standard of care (SOC) and standard practice when determining whether real choice—a prerequisite for SDM—exists in a given medical situation, (2) identifying several areas within the framework that require further specification as elucidated by applying the framework to several hypothetical but representative decision-making scenarios from different pediatric disciplines,[45] and (3) improving the clarity of the framework by adding descriptive titles to each step. Development of the original framework was subjected to iterative critiques by experts in ethics, pediatrics, and medical decision making to help ensure it comprised the key elements of pediatric decision making. The version of the framework presented here represents additional input from a team of investigators with diverse clinical pediatrics backgrounds at Seattle Children's Hospital and at Texas Children's Hospital.

The overall goals of the framework are to increase concordance between parent preferences and implemented interventions as well as to improve medical outcomes for children. The intent is to provide guidance to pediatric clinicians on how and when SDM should be implemented and to provide the foundation and scaffolding for the broad use of SDM across all pediatric disciplines. The framework includes four steps arranged algorithmically (Figure 9.1). Any discrete clinical decision can serve as the starting point. Each of the first three steps poses a question to the physician, with the answers directing the physician further along the algorithm. The last two steps provide guidance on the type and version of SDM that is appropriate to use for the decision under consideration.

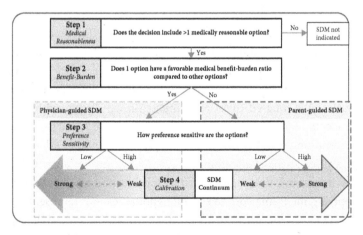

Figure 9.1 Four-step framework for shared decision making (SDM) in pediatrics.

Step 1 (Medical Reasonableness):
Does the Decision Include More Than One
Medically Reasonable Option?

The rationale for this step is that medical situations in which there is only one treatment choice require a different decision-making approach than situations in which several treatment options exist. In the former situation, sharing a decision is not possible because there is no decision to share. Instead, the approach is centered on a discussion with the parent (and when appropriate, the child) about the one available treatment option. Conversely, in the latter situation, the approach does include presenting the several available options and helping the parent choose the option that is aligned with their values.[21] This is the domain of SDM.

Although real choice is a prerequisite for SDM,[21,39,42,46] what constitutes real choice still requires clarification. Some may interpret real choice to mean, for instance, that there is more than one option that represents the SOC, or more than one option that meets a certain threshold of empirical evidence or, perhaps, that is reimbursed. In fact, there are likely myriad factors that might influence what is considered to be a decision with real choice, with some more defensible than others.[33,47] It is also apparent that these factors may not be easily distinguished, such as when value judgments are masqueraded as medical fact.[48,49] Lack of clarity on which factors make up a decision with real choice—and the propensity to conflate them—can have a fundamental influence on the practice of SDM: many decisions that should not be shared with patients are, and those that should be are not.

Some have therefore proposed that "real choice" be defined as "equipoise" in which "options really *are* options."[39] Others have suggested that choice exists in the presence of "reasonable alternatives"[46] or "two or more medically reasonable choices."[42] We propose that real choice exists when there is more than one medically reasonable option, with "medically reasonable" defined as consistent with the SOC.

We have chosen a definition of medically reasonable that is based in the SOC to help ensure what is reasonable at least reflects a consensus basic minimum. Indeed, the SOC requires physicians to provide "minimally competent care" that other physicians would provide under the same circumstances,[50–52] and interventions ideally become the SOC because their safety and efficacy profiles are based upon quality scientific evidence. Professional guideline standards may also help promulgate evidence-based SOC.[53,54] Since physicians who do not practice the SOC risk medical malpractice, negligence, and/or professional discipline, it seems appropriate that what is medically reasonable at least conforms to the SOC.

The Medical Reasonableness step is critical because when there is only one medically reasonable option, SDM is not appropriate. Consider the treatment decision for a child who presents with a moderate acute asthma exacerbation. The combination of short-acting β_2-agonists (SABAs) and corticosteroids is the one medically reasonable option for initial treatment.[55,56] As a result, a non-SDM, physician-controlled approach using a model of simple consent is appropriate.[42] This involves the physician explaining the intervention to the parent (and when appropriate, to the child) followed by a discussion of the intervention's risks and benefits and solicitation of the parent's consent. Discussion of the lack of reasonable alternatives can occur upon parental request. Decisions that exist within this treatment option, such as the type of SABA used (levalbuterol vs. albuterol), should be considered separately, starting with this Medical Reasonableness step.

There are a few anticipated issues with the Medical Reasonableness step that require mention. First, determinations of what is medically reasonable should remain distinct from determinations of the appropriateness of a parent's response to medically reasonable options. For instance, some parents will refuse the one medically acceptable option. Whether or not this refusal is acceptable requires separate consideration (e.g., use of the harm principle to assess whether intervening against parental decision-making authority is justifiable[41]) and will vary by the refusal (e.g., parental refusal of SABA and corticosteroids would likely not be respected, whereas parental refusal of newborn screening—another decision with only one medically reasonable option—would[57]). A non-SDM, physician-controlled decision-making approach, however, is appropriate in both scenarios.

Second, it may be helpful to differentiate SOC from standard practice. As mentioned earlier, the SOC can be legally defined as "minimally competent care." Standard practice is less well defined. In fact, many may consider standard practice to be interchangeable with SOC. However, standard practice can also be considered to be distinct from the SOC as representing an organization's set of criteria for completing a clinical task. In this latter conceptualization, what is standard practice typically aims to meet or exceed the SOC by being "legitimized or validated based on scientific or epidemiological data" and "representing the widely agreed upon, state-of-the-art, high-quality level of practice."[58] Standard practice at an organization can exceed the SOC by including interventions or tests beyond those minimally required based on emerging high-quality data, organizational-level experience, or availability of advanced technologies. It is important for physicians to recognize when standard practice at their organization exceeds the SOC in order to not artificially limit what is considered to be a medically reasonable option: options that don't conform to what is considered to be organizational standard practice may nonetheless be medically reasonable by still conforming to the SOC (Figure 9.2).

Consider the example of an infant born with congenital diaphragmatic hernia (CDH) who underwent successful repair and is preparing for discharge. The surgical team recommends treatment with a proton pump inhibitor (PPI) at home. This recommendation

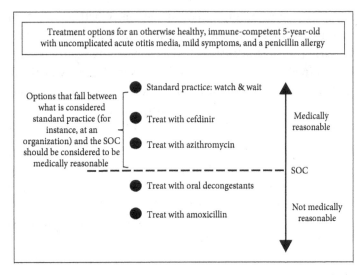

Figure 9.2 Relationship between medically reasonable, standard of care (SOC), and standard practice.

is consistent with an organization's standard practice, is codified in the organization's clinical guidelines, and is based on data illustrating that the majority of infants post-CDH repair develop gastric esophageal reflux (GER).[59] The parents, however, request not starting a PPI to minimize the "medicalization" of their child after such intensive care at the beginning of her life. The surgeons are reluctant to consider this option of no treatment as medically reasonable given that PPI treatment is considered standard practice. However, upon further investigation, they find evidence that defect size is a strong predictor of gastrointestinal morbidity post-CDH repair.[60] This infant had a small defect and is therefore at lower risk of developing GER. Moreover, the child is currently tolerating feeds well and shows no clinical signs of GER. The surgical team therefore correctly determines that while routine treatment with a PPI—the option considered to be standard practice—is medically reasonable, the option to monitor for GER symptoms while off a PPI should also be considered to be a medically reasonable option given supporting evidence that would make it difficult to argue that nontreatment falls below "minimally competent care" (i.e., the SOC).

Third, it can be argued that defining an option as medically reasonable when the SOC is not based on high-quality evidence is problematic. We would agree with this. However, although the ideal is that the SOC be referent only to high-quality, reproducible scientific evidence, there is a practical argument for still considering an option as medically reasonable even though it is based on an SOC composed of low-quality evidence. For instance, this may be the only evidence available, and while not sufficient to serve as a long-term anchor for the SOC, it can serve in this regard temporarily. In addition, maintaining the link of what is medically reasonable to the SOC ensures that the evidence used to justify the SOC meets minimum quality standards. Options based on patient testimonials, opinion polls, or ideology, for instance, are generally excluded because they do not meet the "minimally competent care" requirement.

Fourth, determinations of what is medically reasonable can also be difficult when there is not consensus regarding the SOC. These scenarios are not uncommon in pediatrics: surgical intervention in hypoplastic left heart syndrome[61-63] or trisomy 13[64,65] are two examples. However, it is precisely these scenarios in which there is a lack of consensus that more than one acceptable option likely exists and moving to Step 2 (Benefit-Burden) is warranted.

Lastly, despite this added specificity regarding what constitutes a medically reasonable option, an element of subjectivity remains. Physicians' own biases and values, for instance, may still influence determinations of reasonableness. Furthermore, these factors may wield their influence implicitly under the façade of evidence-based standard practice. Our hope, however, is that this Medical Reasonableness step reduces this subjectivity.

Step 2 (Benefit-Burden): Does One Option Have a Favorable Medical Benefit/Burden Ratio Compared to Other Option(s)?

If a clinical decision includes more than one medically reasonable option, it is appropriate to proceed to Step 2 (Benefit-Burden) to make a reasoned estimation of the ratio of medical benefits and burdens for each option (see Figure 9.1). The rationale for this step is to fulfill physician obligations in pediatrics to ensure that surrogate decisions promote the child's best interests.[40] If one option has a favorable medical benefit-burden ratio compared to other options, it is appropriate for the physician to assume a more directive role in SDM: physician-guided SDM. When there is not a favorable option, it is appropriate to allow the parent to assume a more directive role: parent-guided SDM.

Critical to this step is determining what constitutes a "favorable" option. This involves a judgment based on evidence-based probabilities and magnitudes of the medical benefits and burdens of the options as well as an assessment of the certainty surrounding those probabilities and magnitudes. What balance of probabilities and magnitudes is "favorable" and which benefits and burdens to prioritize in this calculus will likely vary among physicians. Therefore, like the Medical Reasonableness step, this Benefit-Burden step is also susceptible to subjectivity and physician bias. However, this step can help reduce such bias by making these judgments more explicit. For instance, when there is an absence of quality evidence favoring the medical benefit-burden ratio of one option over another, physicians may still make favorability assessments based on their experience or expert opinion but should be aware they are doing so and resist making *strong* favorability judgments.

Another factor to consider when determining the favorability calculus is the physician's dual duty to promote both the public's health and the health and welfare of the patient.[66] As such, this

Benefit-Burden step should include not only benefit-burden assessments relative to the individual child's health but also, where appropriate, benefit-burden assessments relative to the public's health. Consider a scenario in which a child develops hematochezia after eating a hamburger at a fast-food restaurant. She has not developed diarrhea, and on exam, there is an anal fissure present. Since her symptoms began after eating potentially undercooked beef, collecting a stool sample for testing is medically reasonable and may aid in quicker identification of, for example, Shiga toxin–producing *Escherichia coli* as the etiology of her symptoms and the source of an outbreak of food-borne illness. However, watchful waiting also appears to be a medically reasonable option since she doesn't have diarrhea and the blood in her stool could be explained by the anal fissure. In applying the favorability calculus to each option, it seems appropriate to not only consider the individual benefits and burdens of each option (e.g., the cost and inconvenience of testing, the benefit of ruling out a treatable disease with testing) but also the potential benefit to the public of each option (e.g., quicker identification and potential amelioration of an outbreak with testing). The weight that public health considerations deserve compared to those that affect the child's health, however, requires additional analysis.

Step 3 (Preference Sensitivity): How Preference Sensitive Are the Options?

After making a favorability assessment in the Benefit-Burden step, the next step is to determine the parents' preferences regarding the options (see Figure 9.1). The rationale for this step is to ensure parental values and preferences align with the chosen option. In one of the first known descriptions of SDM, the President's Commission acknowledged the importance of "the rights and responsibilities of patients" and proposed SDM as the "ideal for the patient-professional relationship" as medicine shifted away from paternalism.[67]

In situations where there are several medically reasonable options, physicians are obligated to respect the rights and responsibilities of parents by eliciting and incorporating their preferences into decision making. Parents know their child best, are able to weigh competing family interests best, and are allowed to instill in their children the values they have deemed the best.[41] Where options exist—and even when one option appears favorable to the physician—"the best choice depends on how [the parent] values the risks and benefits of the treatments available."[68]

The intent of this Preference Sensitivity step, however, is not to simply elicit what the parent would like to do. Rather, the role of the physician ought to be more expansive and include helping parents articulate their values and preferences: "respecting and responding to patient preferences—the hallmark of patient-centered care— means eliciting, exploring, and questioning preferences and helping patients construct them."[34] Indeed, the ideal physician "is a caring physician who integrates the information and relevant values to make a recommendation and, through discussion, attempts to persuade the patient to accept this recommendation as the intervention that best proposes his or her overall well-being."[18]

The justification for a more expansive physician role in this step is threefold. First, a person's values and preferences—indeed, selfhood—are rarely clear or stable; rather, what one values and prefers is an ongoing process subject to one's capacity for change and reflection. Second, this process is relational: "much of who we are and what we value is rooted in our relationship and affinities with others."[69] It is through our relationships and interactions with others—physicians included—that the development and revision of preferences is facilitated. Third, this more expansive role aligns with the commission's intent for SDM to represent "an appropriate balance" between patient autonomy and a physician's obligation to promote the patient's health and well-being.[67] Simply eliciting parent values and preferences falls short of this balance.

Physicians may feel reluctant to do more than elicit parent preferences. To some, this more expansive role may seem inappropriately intrusive and prone to injecting bias into the decision-making process. The debate surrounding whether and how to answer the patient question "What would you do?" is illustrative,[70–77] as some have argued for a nondirective or value-neutral response to avoid inappropriately influencing the outcome of a preference-sensitive decision.[70,73,76] Our position is that a directive response to this question, particularly after clarifying the parents' intention and disclosing one's own biases and experiences, can support parents in receiving what they desire: help to "clarify relevant values of their own" and which values "should rightly shape such difficult decisions."[77]

This is not to say that physicians ought to coerce, manipulate, or be confrontational with parents or patients. Nor, as the earlier example shows, is it meant to infer that physicians no longer have an obligation to acknowledge and communicate their own preferences. Rather, the Preference Sensitivity step is designed to empower physicians to be involved in helping parents assess the worthiness of certain health-related values and prevent physicians from presuming what parents prefer. Parents may not have a preference between available options despite evidence or experiences suggesting they should (and vice versa); the degree to which preferences matter in a decision may also vary between parents.[78,79] For example, a decision that is not typically preference sensitive, such as which anticoagulant to use to treat a peripherally inserted central catheter–associated thrombus, may be highly preference sensitive to some individuals who wish to avoid porcine-derived products such as heparin due to religious or cultural beliefs. The Preference Sensitivity step helps make explicit what parents prefer and how influential those preferences are to their decision making.

Step 4 (Calibration): Calibrating the Shared Decision-Making Approach

In this last step, we reach a specific SDM approach. Here, SDM is visualized as a continuum, with a physician-guided SDM approach occupying one-half and a parent-guided SDM approach the other (see Figure 9.1). Within each approach there are strong and weak versions, with the strong versions signifying that the parent or physician is appreciably guiding SDM and the weak versions embodying an SDM in which the decision making is more mutual.

To justify the strong version of physician-guided SDM, (1) there must be more than one medically reasonable option for a decision (Step 1, Medical Reasonableness), (2) there must be one option with a favorable medical benefit-burden ratio compared to other options (Step 2, Benefit-Burden), and (3) the favorable option is not preference sensitive (or minimally so) to the parents making the decision (Step 3, Preference Sensitivity). Using a strong version of physician-guided SDM, the physician explains each option and its risks and benefits to ensure the parent is fully informed. The physician then explains that all options are medically appropriate but conveys which option is best based on the physician's reasoned estimation of the medical benefit-burden ratios; subsequently, the physician elicits and helps articulate the parent's preferences. After determining that parental preferences are minimal, the physician seeks explicit parent agreement with the physician-preferred option. If parent preferences change over the course of the discussion, the physician may try to persuade the parent to embrace the values and preferences that align with the physician-preferred option but remains willing to implement the option that is most aligned with parent preferences.

An example in which a strong version of physician-guided SDM may be appropriate is the decision regarding surgical versus medical management in early, uncomplicated appendicitis. Though medical management has emerged as a medically reasonable option to surgical management, the certainty of its risks and benefits is lower compared to surgical management given a paucity of high-quality studies. This, combined with the high efficacy and rare risks with surgical management, makes surgical management the favorable option.[80–82] Use of a strong version of physician-guided SDM, however, would be contingent upon this decision not being very preference sensitive to the parents. If it is clear in the Preference Sensitivity step that this is not the case, a weak version of physician-guided SDM would be indicated. In this weak version, the physician may still try to persuade the parent to embrace the values and preferences that align with the physician-preferred option, but they are more committed to working with the parent to reach a mutual decision aligned with the parent's values and preferences.

To justify the strong version of the parent-guided SDM approach, (1) there must be more than one medically reasonable option for a decision (Step 1, Medical Reasonableness), (2) there must be no favorable option based on medical benefit-burden ratios (Step 2, Benefit-Burden), and (3) the options are very preference sensitive to the parent making the decision (Step 3, Preference Sensitivity). Using a strong version of parent-guided SDM, the physician explains each option and its risks and benefits to ensure the parent is fully informed. The physician explains that each option is medically appropriate and there is no consensus regarding which option is better. In eliciting and helping articulate the parent's preferences, the physician is committed to implementing the intervention that is most closely aligned with the parent's preferences. The physician may make transparent the physician's their preferred option based on their own expertise, experience, and interpretation of the evidence but usually does so only upon parental request.

Male newborn circumcision is illustrative here. Circumcision and no circumcision are both medically reasonable options, and though the medical benefits of circumcision outweigh the risks, "the medical benefits [of circumcision] alone may not outweigh" other considerations to not circumcise, such as religious, cultural, or personal preferences.[83] If circumcision is indeed highly preference sensitive to the particular parents facing this decision, a strong version of parent-guided SDM is appropriate. If it is not very preference sensitive, a weak version of parent-guided SDM is indicated. In this version, the physician still explains that each option is medically appropriate and there is no consensus regarding which option is better, but upon determining that this is not a very preference-sensitive decision to the parents, the physician is more willing to convey the physician's preferred option based on their own expertise, experience, and/or interpretation of the evidence. The physician may even try to persuade the parent to embrace the values and preferences that align with the physician-preferred option but is more committed to working with the parent to reach a mutual decision aligned with the parent's (evolving) values and preferences.

Importantly, this step permits some calibration of SDM based upon the presence of other decisional characteristics besides parent preferences that can shape the SDM approach.[23] These decisional characteristics include the time-sensitiveness or clinical seriousness of the decision, whether the intervention is longitudinal (vs. single event), and whether the intervention is physician (or parent) implemented.[23-27] For instance, longitudinal interventions—such as those that occur in the context of chronic disease (e.g., insulin treatment in diabetes or stimulant medications in attention-deficit/hyperactivity disorder [ADHD])—may calibrate the SDM approach to be more parent guided. This is justified by the need to support more interaction and negotiation as well as maintain compliance in the context of revisiting an intervention over time. Contextual features of the decision may also change over time: patients might get sicker or have adverse effects from prior experiences with the intervention. As such, a strong version of physician-guided SDM may be calibrated to a weaker one or a weak version of parent-guided SDM to a stronger one.

Who implements the intervention may also calibrate the version of SDM used. When parents are primarily responsible for implementation (e.g., supine sleep position or breastfeeding for newborns), SDM should be calibrated to align with this responsibility (i.e., a weaker version of parent-guided SDM can be calibrated to a stronger one). The same is justifiable when physicians are primarily responsible for implementation (i.e., a weak version of physician-guided SDM can be calibrated to a stronger one) to accommodate the particular physician's experience and comfort with the intervention as well as knowledge of unique system-level variables that may influence the success of implementing the intervention in the present clinical setting (e.g., the medically reasonable options to use ketamine or propofol sedation for fracture reduction in the emergency department).

The emotional burden of a decision on parents may also calibrate the SDM approach used given concerns that highly charged emotional states may jeopardize parents' ability to make determinations consistent with their values and preferences, an ability preferred, if not required, for SDM.[84] Consider a young child with a progressive neuromuscular disease who is admitted for respiratory distress. A palliative care physician who knows the family well is asked by the critical care team to discuss the parents' preferences if intubation becomes indicated. The medical team estimates that the child's underlying disease has progressed to the point that he is highly unlikely to tolerate weaning off mechanical ventilation even after recovering from his current viral infection. Thus, for longer-term survival he would likely require a tracheostomy and mechanical ventilation at home. However, the medical team considers intubation or no intubation (with a concomitant focus on the child's comfort as he dies naturally from his underlying incurable illness) as both medically reasonable options. In the past, the child's parents consistently stated that the burdens of mechanical ventilation at home outweighed its benefits and that dependency on a machine is not the quality of life they would want for their child. However, at admission, the parents now state they feel unable to bear the weight of deciding if their child should live or die if intubation is indicated. Though a strong version of parent-guided SDM might be indicated in this case given multiple medically reasonable options that are highly preference sensitive and none of which have a clearly favorable benefit-burden ratio, it may be appropriate to use a weak version of parent-guided SDM given the presence of intense emotions that may impact the parents' ability to participate in SDM. For instance, the physician, repeating back the parents' previously stated values, could make a recommendation to the parents that respiratory support be provided up to the point of intubation, but no further. The physician could then ask if this still fits with the parents' values and preferences or if their opinions have since evolved.

The Calibration step builds upon Kon's model for SDM[38] by incorporating additional variables beyond parent preferences to calibrate SDM. Though the examples provided previously are intended to provide some guidance on how these variables can influence the SDM approach used, this is still an area of active inquiry. For instance, variables may impose opposite pressures on how SDM is calibrated, such as in scenarios involving longitudinal but physician-implemented interventions (e.g., childhood immunizations). Whether these variables are canceling or should be weighted differently requires additional analyses.

Conclusion

We have described a framework for when and how to implement SDM in pediatrics. These steps and the justifications therein can help ensure that SDM is used appropriately and accounts for the decisional and contextual features unique to pediatrics. The overall goals of the framework are to increase concordance between parent preferences and implemented interventions as well as to improve medical outcomes for children. Although additional analyses are needed to consider the limitations of each of these steps, the framework can function as a foundation and scaffolding for the broad use of SDM across all pediatric disciplines.

Acknowledgments

The authors thank Katherine Lepere, BA; Doug Diekema, MD, MPH; Ben Wilfond, MD; Seema Shah, JD; Abby Rosenberg, MD; Elliott Weiss, MD; Jon Tilburt, MD; Mara Buchbinder, PhD; Neal Dickert, MD; Jennifer Blumenthal-Barby, PhD; Amy McGuire, JD; and Bernie Lo, MD, for their comments on the original version of this framework. We also thank Emily Kroshus, PhD; Jonna Clark, MD; Carrie Heike, MD; and Laura Loftis, MD, for their input on subsequent refinements to the original framework.

References

1. Barry MJ, Edgman-Levitan S. Shared decision making—pinnacle of patient-centered care. *N Engl J Med*. 2012;366(9):780–781.
2. Charles C, Gafni A, Whelan T. Shared decision-making in the medical encounter: what does it mean? (or it takes at least two to tango). *Soc Sci Med (1982)*. 1997;44(5):681–692.
3. Jonsen AR. *The Birth of Bioethics*. New York: Oxford University Press; 1998.
4. Schloendorff v. Society of New York Hospital. 211 N.Y. 125, 105 N.E. 92 1914.
5. Salgo v. Leland Stanford Jr. University Board of Trustees. 317 P.2d 170 (Cal. Ct. App. 1957) 1957.
6. Canterbury v. Spence. U.S. Court of Appeals for the District of Columbia Circuit 464 F.2d 772 (D.C. Cir. 1972) 1972.
7. Stacey D, Legare F, Lewis KB. Patient decision aids to engage adults in treatment or screening decisions. *JAMA*. 2017;318(7):657–658.
8. Braddock CH 3rd. Supporting shared decision making when clinical evidence is low. *Med Care Res Rev MCRR*. 2013;70(1 Suppl):129S–140S.
9. Frosch DL, Kaplan RM. Shared decision making in clinical medicine: past research and future directions. *Am J Prevent Med*. 1999;17(4):285–294.
10. Montori VM, Kunneman M, Brito JP. Shared decision making and improving health care: the answer is not in. *JAMA*. 2017; 318(7):617–618.

11. Gartner FR, Bomhof-Roordink H, Smith IP, Scholl I, Stiggelbout AM, Pieterse AH. The quality of instruments to assess the process of shared decision making: a systematic review. *PLoS One*. 2018;13(2):e0191747.

12. Shay LA, Lafata JE. Where is the evidence? A systematic review of shared decision making and patient outcomes. *Med Decis Making*. 2015;35(1):114–131.

13. Stacey D, Legare F, Lewis K, et al. Decision aids for people facing health treatment or screening decisions. *Cochrane Database Syst Rev*. 2017;4:CD001431.

14. Brock DW. The ideal of shared decision making between physicians and patients. *Kennedy Inst Ethics J*. 1991;1(1):28–47.

15. Quill TE, Brody H. Physician recommendations and patient autonomy: finding a balance between physician power and patient choice. *Ann Intern Med*. 1996;125(9):763–769.

16. Veatch RM. Modern vs. contemporary medicine: the patient-provider relation in the twenty-first century. *Kennedy Inst Ethics J*. 1996;6(4):366–370.

17. Katz J. *The Silent World of Doctor and Patient*. Baltimore, MD: Johns Hopkins University Press; 2002.

18. Emanuel EJ, Emanuel LL. Four models of the physician-patient relationship. *JAMA*. 1992;267(16):2221–2226.

19. Fried TR. Shared decision making—finding the sweet spot. *N Engl J Med*. 2016;374(2):104–106.

20. Rosenbaum L. The paternalism preference—choosing unshared decision making. *N Engl J Med*. 2015;373(7):589–592.

21. Whitney SN, Holmes-Rovner M, Brody H, et al. Beyond shared decision making: an expanded typology of medical decisions. *Med Decis Making*. 2008;28(5):699–705.

22. Sandman L, Munthe C. Shared decision making, paternalism and patient choice. *Health Care Anal*. 2010;18(1):60–84.

23. Montori VM, Gafni A, Charles C. A shared treatment decision-making approach between patients with chronic conditions and their clinicians: the case of diabetes. *Health Expect*. 2006;9(1):25–36.

24. Weiss EM, Barg FK, Cook N, Black E, Joffe S. Parental decision-making preferences in neonatal intensive care. *J Pediatr*. 2016;179:36–41.e33.

25. Muller-Engelmann M, Keller H, Donner-Banzhoff N, Krones T. Shared decision making in medicine: the influence of situational treatment factors. *Patient Educ Couns*. 2011;82(2):240–246.

26. Kaplan RM. Shared medical decision making. A new tool for preventive medicine. *Am J Prevent Med*. 2004;26(1):81–83.

27. Keirns CC, Goold SD. Patient-centered care and preference-sensitive decision making. *JAMA*. 2009;302(16):1805–1806.

28. Opel DJ. A push for progress with shared decision-making in pediatrics. *Pediatrics*. 2017;139(2):e20162526.

29. Aronson PL, Fraenkel L. Is shared decision-making the right approach for febrile infants? *Pediatrics*. 2017;140(3):e20170225.

30. Birchley G. Deciding together? Best interests and shared decision-making in paediatric intensive care. *Health Care Anal*. 2014;22(3):203–222.

31. Gillam L, Wilkinson D, Xafis V, Isaacs D. Decision-making at the borderline of viability: who should decide and on what basis? *J Paediatr Child Health*. 2017;53(2):105–111.

32. Tilburt J. Shared decision making after MacIntyre. *J Med Philos*. 2011;36(2):148–169.

33. Wirtz V, Cribb A, Barber N. Patient-doctor decision-making about treatment within the consultation—a critical analysis of models. *Soc Sci Med*. 2006;62(1):116–124.

34. Epstein RM, Peters E. Beyond information: exploring patients' preferences. *JAMA*. 2009;302(2):195–197.

35. Whitney SN. A new model of medical decisions: exploring the limits of shared decision making. *Med Decis Making*. 2003;23(4):275–280.

36. Murray E, Charles C, Gafni A. Shared decision-making in primary care: tailoring the Charles et al. model to fit the context of general practice. *Patient Educ Couns*. 2006;62(2):205–211.

37. Murray E, Pollack L, White M, Lo B. Clinical decision-making: patients' preferences and experiences. *Patient Educ Couns*. 2007;65(2):189–196.

38. Kon AA. The shared decision-making continuum. *JAMA*. 2010;304(8):903–904.

39. Gwyn R, Elwyn G. When is a shared decision not (quite) a shared decision? Negotiating preferences in a general practice encounter. *Soc Sci Med (1982)*. 1999;49(4):437–447.

40. Beauchamp T, Childress J. *Principles of Biomedical Ethics*. 5th ed. New York: Oxford University Press; 2001.

41. Diekema DS. Parental refusals of medical treatment: the harm principle as threshold for state intervention. *Theor Med Bioeth*. 2004;25(4):243–264.

42. Whitney SN, McGuire AL, McCullough LB. A typology of shared decision making, informed consent, and simple consent. *Ann Intern Med*. 2003;140(1):54–59.

43. Elwyn G, Frosch D, Thomson R, et al. Shared decision making: a model for clinical practice. *J Gen Intern Med*. 2012;27(10):1361–1367.

44. Opel DJ. A 4-step framework for shared decision-making in pediatrics. *Pediatrics*. 2018;142(Suppl 3):S149–S156.

45. Weiss EM, Clark JD, Heike CL, et al. Gaps in the implementation of shared decision-making: illustrative. *Pediatrics*. 2019;In press.

46. Elwyn G, Frosch DL, Kobrin S. Implementing shared decision-making: consider all the consequences. *Implement Sci*. 2016;11:114. doi:10.1186/213012-016-0480-9.

47. Sculpher M, Gafni A, Watt I. Shared treatment decision making in a collectively funded health care system: possible conflicts and some potential solutions. *Soc Sci Med.* 2002;54(9):1369–1377.

48. Opel DJ, Taylor JA, Phillipi CA, Diekema DS. The intersection of evidence and values in clinical guidelines: who decides what constitutes acceptable risk in the care of children? *Hosp Pediatr.* 2013;3(2):87–91.

49. Ubel PA. Medical facts versus value judgments—toward preference-sensitive guidelines. *N Engl J Med.* 2015;372(26):2475–2477.

50. Hall v. Hilburn. 466 S. 2d 856 (Miss. 1985).

51. McCourt v. Abernathy. 457 S.E.2d 603 (S.C. 1995).

52. Johnston v. St. Francis Medical Center, Inc. No. 3–5, 236-CA, Oct. 31, 2001.

53. Institute of Medicine, Committee on Standards for Developing Trustworthy Clinical Practice Guidelines, Board on Health Care Services. *Clinical Practice Guidelines We Can Trust.* Washington, DC: National Academies Press; 2011.

54. Guyatt GH, Oxman AD, Vist GE, et al. GRADE: an emerging consensus on rating quality of evidence and strength of recommendations. *BMJ Clin Res.* 2008;336(7650):924–926.

55. Castro-Rodriguez JA, Rodrigo JG, Rodriguez-Martinez CE. Principal findings of systematic reviews of acute asthma treatment in childhood. *J Asthma.* 2015;52(10):1038–1045.

56. Okpapi A, Friend AJ, Turner SW. Asthma and other recurrent wheezing disorders in children (acute). *BMJ Clin Evid.* 2012;2012:0300. https://pubmed.ncbi.nlm.nih.gov/22305975/. Accessed April 28, 2021.

57. American Academy of Pediatrics Committee on Bioethics, Committee on Genetics, and, the American College of Medical Genetics, and Genomics Social, Ethical, and Legal Issues Committee. Ethical and policy issues in genetic testing and screening of children. *Pediatrics.* 2013;131(3):620–622.

58. American Academy of Pediatrics. Definitions Explained: Standards, Recommendations, Guidelines, and Regulations. 2017. https://www.aap.org/en-us/Documents/Definitions_StandardsGuidelines.pdf. Accessed February 12, 2019.

59. Su W, Berry M, Puligandla PS, Aspirot A, Flageole H, Laberge JM. Predictors of gastroesophageal reflux in neonates with congenital diaphragmatic hernia. *J Pediatr Surg.* 2007;42(10):1639–1643.

60. Putnam LR, Harting MT, Tsao K, et al. Congenital diaphragmatic hernia defect size and infant morbidity at discharge. *Pediatrics.* 2016;138(5):e20162043.

61. Feudtner C. Ethics in the midst of therapeutic evolution. *Arch Pediatr Adolesc Med.* 2008;162(9):854–857.

62. Kon AA. Healthcare providers must offer palliative treatment to parents of neonates with hypoplastic left heart syndrome. *Arch Pediatr Adolesc Med.* 2008;162(9):844–848.

63. Wernovsky G. The paradigm shift toward surgical intervention for neonates with hypoplastic left heart syndrome. *Arch Pediatr Adolesc Med.* 2008;162(9):849–854.

64. Nelson KE, Rosella LC, Mahant S, Guttmann A. Survival and surgical interventions for children with trisomy 13 and 18. *JAMA.* 2016;316(4):420–428.

65. Lantos JD. Trisomy 13 and 18—treatment decisions in a stable gray zone. *JAMA.* 2016;316(4):396–398.

66. American Medical Association. *Code of Medical Ethics: Physicians and the Health of the Community.* Chicago, IL: AMA Press; 2016.

67. President's Commission for the Study of Ethical Problems in Medicine and Biomedical and Behavioral Research. *Making Health Care Decisions: A Report on the Ethical and Legal Implications of Informed Consent in the Patient-Practitioner Relationship.* Washington, DC: US Government Printing Office; 1982.

68. Elwyn G, Frosch D, Rollnick S. Dual equipoise shared decision making: definitions for decision and behaviour support interventions. *Implement Sci.* 2009;4:75.

69. Sherwin S. *The Politics of Women's Health: Exploring Agency and Autonomy in Health Care.* Philadelphia: Temple University Press; 1998.

70. Gutgesell HP. What if it were your child? *Am J Cardiol.* 2002;89(7):856.

71. Truog R. Revisiting "Doctor, if this were your child, what would you do?" *J Clin Ethics.* 2003;14(1–2):63–67.

72. Halpern J. Responding to the need behind the question "Doctor, if this were your child, what would you do?" *J Clin Ethics.* 2003;14(1–2):71–78.

73. Ruddick W. Answering parents' questions. *J Clin Ethics.* 2003;14(1–2):68–70.

74. Ross LF. Why "doctor, if this were your child, what would you do?" deserves an answer. *J Clin Ethics.* 2003;14(1–2):59–62.

75. Kon AA. Answering the question: "Doctor, if this were your child, what would you do?" *Pediatrics.* 2006;118(1):393–397.

76. Truog RD. "Doctor, if this were your child, what would you do?" *Pediatrics.* 1999;103(1):153–154.

77. Tucker Edmonds B, Torke AM, Helft P, Wocial LD. Doctor, what would you do? an answer for patients requesting advice about value-laden decisions. *Pediatrics.* 2015;136(4):740–745.

78. Madrigal VN, Carroll KW, Hexem KR, Faerber JA, Morrison WE, Feudtner C. Parental decision-making preferences in the pediatric intensive care unit. *Crit Care Med.* 2012;40(10):2876–2882.

79. Tom DM, Aquino C, Arredondo AR, Foster BA. Parent preferences for shared decision-making in acute versus chronic illness. *Hosp Pediatr.* 2017;7(10):602–609.
80. Huang L, Yin Y, Yang L, Wang C, Li Y, Zhou Z. Comparison of antibiotic therapy and appendectomy for acute uncomplicated appendicitis in children: a meta-analysis. *JAMA Pediatr.* 2017;171(5):426–434.
81. Lopez ME, Wesson DE. Medical treatment of pediatric appendicitis: are we there yet? *JAMA Pediatr.* 2017;171(5):419–420.
82. Bachur RG, Rangel SJ. The threat of diagnostic uncertainty in the medical management of uncomplicated appendicitis. *JAMA Pediatr.* 2017;171(6):505–506.
83. American Academy of Pediatrics Task Force on Circumcision. Male circumcision. *Pediatrics.* 2012;130(3):e756–785.
84. Rosenberg AR, Dussel V, Kang T, et al. Psychological distress in parents of children with advanced cancer. *JAMA Pediatr.* 2013;167(6):537–543.

10

Cross-Cultural Interactions and Shared Decision Making

Sabrina F. Derrington and Erin Paquette

If you have come here to help me, you are wasting your time. But if you have come because your liberation is bound up with mine, then let us work together.

—Activist, academic, and artist Lilla Watson

Introduction

This chapter explores the interplay between culture and shared decision making (SDM), highlighting cases in which cultural differences may impact decision making and suggesting recommendations for optimizing cultural humility in all aspects of communication and SDM. We focus on pediatric cases, but our conceptual framework would apply equally to cases involving adults.

Culture can have a significant impact on the SDM process. Because SDM relies on a robust understanding of the patient/family's goals, preferences, values, and beliefs, assumptions about what is known, understood, or prioritized can undermine the process. Assumptions and stereotypes occur more frequently when cultural differences are present, and are even more likely to be incomplete or frankly incorrect.[1-3] Education that encourages avoiding stereotypes and awareness of bias and that conceptualizes culture as part of one's moral experience may avoid these difficulties.[4-6]

The Many Facets of Culture

Broadly defined, culture reflects the "shared values, beliefs, and behaviors by which people interpret life's events."[7] Interpretation of self and others necessarily involves interaction, and culture, therefore, is also defined by shared communication and interpretation. This definition encompasses the breadth of culture that may impact decision making, which spans more than the narrow conceptualization of culture often described by programs teaching "cultural competency" as related to race, ethnicity, language, and religion. Culture in health care decision making includes many additional considerations including, among others, family traditions, the culture of medicine, perceptions of illness and death, socioeconomic status, geography, and education.

The following case-based approach illustrates some of the challenges that can arise with cultural differences during SDM in the pediatric intensive care unit (PICU). Where necessary, names and any identifying features have been altered.

Culture and Race/Ethnicity

The well-known case of Jahi McMath involved an adolescent who was declared brain dead following complications from a tonsillectomy. The family rejected the declaration of brain death, and while much discussion of the case focused on the meaning of death and brain death, several ethicists examining the case have noted the role of race in the family's interactions with the medical team and their refusal to allow withdrawal of the ventilator following the determination of brain death. In discussions about their daughter following her death, comments such as "If Jahi was a little White girl, I feel we would have gotten a little more help and attention" and "Do you think we're supposed to be used to our children dying, that this is just what Black people normally go through?" highlight the perception of the family that race influenced the care she received and how the family should view the situation.[8]

Race and ethnicity, like religion, are traditionally thought of as framing one's culture and often form the basis of "cultural competency" training. However, learning broad generalizations about particular groups can lead to stereotyping and actually cause more harm than good. There is more to be gained by teaching cultural humility—which recognizes race and ethnicity as a small part of an individual's multifaceted cultural identity.[9]

Race and ethnicity play an important and independent role in shared medical decision making, in large part because of the longstanding history of institutionalized racism and discrimination in this country. As the McMath case demonstrated, even if it was not recognized by the news media or the bioethics community when Jahi's story first became public, her family perceived their interactions with the medical team and the hospital to be impacted by their race. There are complex interactions between patients' race/ethnicity and their socioeconomic class and education, which affect the health information they receive, their confidence in that information, and their trust in the health system. Richardson et al. found that individuals of lower socioeconomic status as marked by education level and income were less likely to seek health information and less confident in the information they received, while individuals of racial and ethnic minorities as well as those of lower income had lower trust in doctors and the health system when seeking health information.[10]

Adequate information exchange is essential to optimizing SDM. Medical providers should be aware of the potential impact of cultural factors during their communication with patients and families. Consideration of the influence of race/ethnicity on perceptions around communication may be particularly important when discussing end-of-life care. Harris et al. showed that families from racial/ethnic minorities pursued more aggressive end-of-life care, while Lee et al. showed that families of racial/ethnic minorities reported lower perceptions of the quality of their loved one's death.[11,12] While there is insufficient evidence to evaluate the influence of race/ethnicity on parental decision making, providers should be sensitive to the ways in which racial/ethnic identity is present in all decision making, and further research should aim to address these knowledge gaps.

Culture and Religion

Jacob is a 9-year-old previously healthy boy who was found floating in a neighbor's pool, unconscious, not breathing, and without a pulse. After nearly 30 minutes of cardiopulmonary resuscitation (CPR) he was stabilized and admitted to the PICU. After 2 days of full physiologic support brain death testing was performed, Jacob demonstrated no brainstem reflexes, but during the apnea test he initiated several ragged breaths. The PICU team explained to the family that Jack had sustained irreversible, devastating brain injury and recommended withdrawal of mechanical ventilation to allow a peaceful death. They also explained that, if they wanted to prolong Jacob's life, he would need a tracheostomy and long-term ventilation, as well as a feeding tube. Jacob's parents listened tearfully with heads bowed, then looked up and quietly said, "Doctor, we respect your expertise, but we are people of faith, and we believe in miracles. We know that God is going to heal Jacob. We are going to fast and pray, and we'd like to bring our minister in to perform a healing." They refused to consider a tracheostomy and feeding tube because they did not think it would be necessary, and they requested that Jacob remain a "full code."

Many parents of seriously ill children and family members of seriously ill adults incorporate spiritual and religious beliefs into medical decision making. They rely on faith and spirituality as important sources of emotional coping.[13,14] But these beliefs are seldom discussed. There are many reasons for the silence. Not all parents want physicians to inquire about their religious or spiritual beliefs. Even among parents who want their physicians to know about their religious and spiritual beliefs, a minority bring up the topic themselves.[15] Physicians are unlikely to elicit a spiritual history. This mutual discomfort in discussing religion and spirituality contributes to breakdowns in the SDM process as conflict around a difficult decision might be the first time that crucial religious or spiritual beliefs are shared.

In general, physicians are less likely than the general public to claim a personal religious identity or to describe themselves as "very spiritual."[16,17] Health care providers may thus be likely to hold different beliefs than those held by patients and families.[18] Medical providers may be dismissive of religious values that are at odds with medical recommendations. In addition, reliance on stereotypes of religious or spiritual traditions is a potential pitfall for SDM. The impact of patient/family religion and spirituality on medical decision making varies widely even within a specific religion and cannot be assumed or anticipated based on demographics.[19,20]

Even if Jacob's parents had not previously shared information about their religious beliefs, their faith in God is playing a central role in their current decision making, functioning in both positive and negative ways. For example, belief in God's supernatural power and control over the world may be helping them cope with a horrible prognosis and the limits of medicine, while allowing them to postpone acceptance of a harsh new reality. Their health care team will need to continue engaging with them in a way that acknowledges and supports this important source of coping, while employing strategies and frameworks from within their worldview to facilitate acceptance and decision making.[20] Partnering with spiritual care providers, including the family's minister as well as the hospital chaplain, may be an important part of that journey.

Culture and Tradition

Abeo was a 5-month-old male dying from complications of a serious infection. The child's dedicated family had been constantly at his bedside, talking to him, deeply hopeful about recovery but also understanding and accepting of updates from the team when he deteriorated. After several conversations about his high probability of decompensation, the family was in agreement with the medical team to optimize comfort, withdraw life-sustaining therapies, and allow a peaceful death. When this decision was made, the family began to walk out of the room, indicating that they must remember the child alive, and could not be present for his death. They asked the medical team to ensure that their child was not alone at the end. The bedside staff were entirely supportive of the family's perspective and remained with the baby until he died.

Culture and traditions are inextricably linked. With respect to health care decision making, traditions within cultures may have an impact across many decisions and practices. Among others, key areas in which tradition may impact SDM include decisions about who is the primary decision maker or spokesperson for a family, feeding/personal care, end-of-life care, and death itself.

Decision Maker/Communication

In many cultures patriarchal figures are the primary communicators and decision makers for their families, grounded in social structures and traditions.[3] This traditional role sometimes dictates that they protect other family members or the patient themselves by hiding certain medical information from them, creating moral distress among a care team. Although Western medicine favors transparency for optimal decision making, practicing with cultural humility should prompt sensitive inquiry about a family's culture and traditions. This may include reaching out to others who practice similar religious or social traditions to obtain insight about these cultural influences and to discern a path forward that honors the patient's culture and traditions while ensuring appropriate respect for their personhood.

Feeding

Similarly, cultural traditions may impact how families respond to decisions about providing artificial nutrition to their loved ones. Whether rooted in religion or in nonreligious social practices, diverse cultures may have different levels of acceptance for the provision of any artificial nutrition or hydration (enteral or parenteral) and for withdrawing artificial nutrition/hydration once it has been initiated.[21-23] This may lead to tensions around placement of feeding tubes or central lines, the actual provision of nutrition, what kind of nutrition is provided, and whether or when to stop artificial nutrition and hydration. As feeding patients using artificial means is a medical intervention, patients and their surrogates must provide consent, and attention to their cultural traditions will be important in the SDM process.

Dying

In Abeo's case earlier cultural traditions around death precluded the family's presence at the bedside when their child died. While this was a departure from how the majority might respond in both the medical culture and good-parent culture (see later), the medical team in his case was able to accommodate their beliefs to support the family. Traditions around end-of-life care, the process of dying, and death itself are deeply influenced by culture and its interplay with faith, religion, and values.[24] Family willingness to discuss advanced care planning may be influenced by how much they are traditionally willing to discuss their child's medical condition among the decision makers and with the child.[3,25] Willingness to engage with palliative care may be similarly impacted by cultural traditions or beliefs around communication and perceptions of suffering, death, and dying. At the time of death, families may be unable to decline or may request interventions that the medical team feels are inappropriate because of cultural expectations that "everything was done."[26,27] Similarly, they may request certain traditions or rituals be performed as part of the dying process.[26] The complex interplay between many facets of death and dying may also place one in multiple cultures, requiring providers to be attuned to the specific context of the patient and family, who may be situated in many cultures.[28]

Medical Cultures

The Good-Parent Culture

Mateo was a 3-year-old patient with relapsed leukemia who required stem cell transplantation and whose posttransplant course was complicated by multiple life-threatening episodes and intractable pain that ultimately prompted his medical team to recommend withdrawal of life-sustaining therapies to his parents. The team felt strongly that the family would struggle with decision making and made a strong recommendation for withdrawal of life-sustaining therapies with allowance of a peaceful death, permitting the parents to agree by nondissent.[29] His parents, who were in their early 20s, Spanish-speaking, and often felt by the medical team to be detached from their son, rejected the recommendation, passionately expressing a desire to "not give up." The team agreed to continue current support; gradually Mateo weaned from multiple intensive interventions and was eventually transferred to rehabilitation with tracheostomy but no ventilator, and with his parent's active engagement.

Pediatric providers tend to have specific expectations of parents of sick children. Good parents are at their child's bedside much of the time, are present for family-centered rounds, are available for medical updates or informed consent conversations, ask thoughtful questions, and respect our expert opinions. In this sense, we create cultural norms for parents of a sick child, and we struggle when parents do not demonstrate behaviors consistent with our expectations, often failing to recognize or sympathize with the many reasons that parents might not conform to the "parent of a sick child" culture. For example, Mateo's parents might have been afraid to touch him or stand too close to all his tubes and machines; they might have worried that their expression of emotion would be perceived as weakness. And in the care conference they demonstrated their own, different beliefs around what it means to be a good parent to a sick child: not giving up, advocating for ongoing support, and waiting patiently for the recovery that eventually came.[30]

The Sick-Patient Culture

In the *Private Worlds of Dying Children*, Myra Blue-Bond Langner writes about the culture of patients in the hospital from the standpoint of children:

> For example, Faith (age three) interpreted the hospital as a threatening place. Those associated with it, inflicted pain. Whenever anyone in white approached Faith, she dove under the covers. Jeffrey (age five), like Faith, saw the hospital in terms of "us" and "them." He made his primary cut . . . on the basis of those in uniform vs those not in uniform. He later moved to a more behavioral based interpretation—those who took orders and spoke only when spoken to versus those who came and went when they pleased, sometimes with and sometimes without explanation, a practice usually reserved for adults. On the basis of these

interpretations, Jeffrey refrained from questioning the medical staff about his condition and assumed a supplicant position.[31]

A child's experience of illness itself is shaped by social and cultural influences.[32] Some illnesses may be shaped by how a society or cultural framework views their illness, influencing their experiences of illness. One's understanding of their illness is also shaped by their cultural influences. Their knowledge of illness may also be socially constructed on some level, impacted by the medical culture (see later) and parent or family beliefs.[33] In this "sick patient" culture, some may choose not to disclose information to a child perceived as vulnerable. How much information a child directly or indirectly receives influences their ability to participate in decision making and may alter their experience.[34] For chronically critically ill children or children facing life-limiting illness, the culture of the hospital around them can create a positive or negative illness experience.[35] Recognizing the interplay between the illness culture and hospital culture to meet the needs of patients and families may improve decision making in both day-to-day decisions and larger decisions around goals of care.[36]

The Culture(s) of Medicine

It is important to acknowledge that medicine has a culture of its own, with deeply ingrained values and beliefs that may be quite different from those of patients and families. For example, Western medicine tends to value inductive rather than deductive reasoning, empiric rather than anecdotal evidence, and rational rather than emotional decision making. The focus is on addressing the physical aspects of disease using pharmacologic, interventional, and technological therapies, often neglecting the psychosocial, emotional, and spiritual components of illness.[37] These biases influence the expectations that providers have of patients and families engaged in an SDM process.

Equally relevant are the cultural differences that exist between medical specialties and disciplines. Group perspectives, priorities, and behavioral norms may affect interactions with members of other groups within the health care team and can also impact patients and families. For example, while some overlap exists, nurses and physicians identify different ethical concerns in end-of-life care decisions and experience different sources of moral distress.[38-40] Among physicians from different specialties, variations have been documented in perceptions of patient and family needs, such as readiness to discuss palliative care, and in physician communication and decision-making styles.[41-43] For health care providers, acknowledging one's own assumptions and biases pertaining to the culture of the discipline, specialty, or institution and cultivating awareness of the different perspectives, ethical sensitivities, and professional practices of other health care team members are essential to safe, effective patient care—and to the often multidisciplinary nature of SDM.

Culture Between Provider and Patient/Family

Cultural differences between health care providers and the patients and families they serve can threaten the delicate process of SDM in multiple ways. For instance, providers and patients/families may make assumptions or rely on stereotypes of unfamiliar cultures in an attempt to understand each other, but these interpretations are highly likely to be incomplete or even completely wrong.[3] Even providers who eschew stereotypes may hold implicit (subconscious) biases that influence the way they present medical information and even the extent of information provided.[44] On the other hand, patients/families may also be subject to implicit or explicit bias, or they may have prior experiences of discrimination (personally or culturally) that contribute to distrust, misperception, and misunderstanding.[45]

Communication of complex medical information and eliciting patient/family values and goals are difficult when a language barrier exists. Differences between provider and patient/family, whether in ethnicity, race, language, religion, or socioeconomic class, make difficult conversations even more uncomfortable. In a study of over 1,000 physicians of different specialties caring for diverse, seriously ill patients, doctors reported multiple barriers to end-of-life conversations with patients of other ethnicities, most notably language differences; patient/family religio-spiritual beliefs about death and dying; doctors' ignorance of patients' cultural beliefs, values, and practices; cultural differences in truth handling and decision making; patients' limited health literacy; and patients' mistrust of doctors and the health care system.[46]

The Impact of Culture

Culturally Based Refusals

Cultural differences may lead families to refuse interventions that the medical team feels are essential for a patient, or to refuse to stop interventions that the medical team believes are harmful for a patient. In the first situation, the refusal raises questions of medical neglect, while in the second, it raises questions of futility.[47] Such refusals create conflict between the medical team and the family and impede SDM. Refusals of care in pediatrics are challenging because of the fiduciary responsibility of health care providers to protect the best interests of a child and provide for the child's future autonomy, and because of the pediatrician's role as a mandated reporter when they believe that a parent's medical decision rises to the level of abuse or neglect of a child.[48]

Culturally based refusals are often tied to claims of deeply held religious beliefs or cultural traditions. Common refusals include the refusal to place a feeding tube or means for nutrition/hydration in cultures that do not support artificial nutrition and the refusal to withdraw or withhold invasive interventions at end of life while "waiting for a miracle." Recently, families have increasingly rejected or refused the diagnosis of brain death, with cultural considerations playing at least a partial role in the refusal.[8] Conflict can arise when teams challenge the legitimacy of these beliefs; hold different, irreconcilable religious beliefs themselves; or believe that the reliance on these beliefs leads a child to suffer harm from interventions that are invasive or unlikely to succeed.[49,50]

Managing cultural-based refusals is a challenge for medical teams. Initially, such refusals should be approached in the same manner as any disagreement between the medical team and family. Frameworks such as those suggested to deal with disagreements over "potentially inappropriate care," including the use of family meetings, conflict resolution principles, and family engagement, are important. Discussions with the family should incorporate explicit consideration of their cultural beliefs and preferences, including their preferences for receiving information, eliciting information about their religious or spiritual beliefs, and inquiry into their cultural practices or traditions.[51] When family preferences for care raise concerns about pain or suffering, attempts at respectful negotiation should be undertaken, unless decisions rise to the level of abuse or neglect. Involving state actors to consider abuse or neglect claims should be a last resort, particularly in the setting of cultural differences between a family and medical team, which are likely to also be present between state actors and the family. At critical points in illness, state involvement is also likely to further fragment relationships with families who may already be distrustful, may create administrative delays in decision making for the child, and will likely further strain a family that is already experiencing significant stress. Although the best-interest standard guides medical decision making for children and is what medical teams and parents should use as a guiding principle in their decisions, medical teams may turn to the harm principle to guide when state action may be necessary. This principle suggests that the state should only be involved when family decisions pose a risk of substantial harm or death.[52] If medical teams are adhering to principles of cultural humility and SDM, it is unlikely that state involvement will be necessary.

Culture and Health Disparities

Disparities between different racial/ethnic, socioeconomic, and linguistic groups have been thoroughly documented in the literature for a wide range of health outcomes. While many of these differences are tied to health care access, cultural differences between providers and patients/families that disrupt SDM and compromise communication lead to lower-quality care and worse outcomes. SDM requires communication skills, not just in sharing information but also in eliciting patient/family values and preferences. Providers with higher levels of implicit bias (pro-White, anti-Black) tend to spend more time talking and less time listening and have more dominant communication styles and lower levels of patient-perceived collaboration in racially discordant interactions.[53] Nonverbal communication behaviors, so important in building rapport and demonstrating compassion, are demonstrated less frequently by physicians interacting with Black patients, even in discussions about end-of-life treatment decisions.[54] It is no wonder, then, that African American cancer patients in the Coping with Cancer study were more likely than White patients to receive aggressive, life-prolonging interventions, regardless of their expressed preferences.[55]

Non-English-speaking patients and families also experience poor communication and worse health outcomes, but a limited body of literature suggests that this problem is one that can be addressed. Anand et al. found that Latino children admitted to their tertiary care PICU had a 3.7-fold higher odds of mortality compared to White children but that after a multilevel, multidisciplinary intervention to implement culturally and linguistically sensitive care, that difference disappeared.[56]

Limited English proficiency and low health literacy present two separate but overlapping disadvantages that contribute to poor health outcomes for adult and pediatric patients.[57] Careful assessment of health literacy, as well as individual values and beliefs around health, illness, and death, is necessary to facilitate SDM and advance care planning.[58]

Vulnerable patient groups may be at heightened disadvantage in the unfamiliar hospital culture. Especially in the context of rare, life-threatening diseases, parents' ability to navigate the health care system and the hospital/medical team hierarchy, to advocate for their child in the most effective way possible, may become a matter of life or death.[59]

Ethical Frameworks and Culturally Sensitive Communication

Several ethical frameworks are relevant to incorporating cultural humility into SDM. Traditional ethical principles of autonomy, beneficence, nonmaleficence, and justice are all implicated. Autonomy is relevant to any decision-making situation, including by surrogates. To fully respect autonomy, relevant information must be communicated in a culturally sensitive manner and with enough knowledge of the decision maker's relevant values and beliefs to ensure they can exercise an authentic choice. Practicing with cultural humility also respects the principle of nonmaleficence by avoiding the psychological harm that can accompany miscommunication or discrimination. Promoting authentic decision making will likely result in the decision that is best for the patient, supporting benef-icence. Working to eliminate disparities that may exist due to cul-tural differences promotes justice.

However, some have criticized the four-principles approach as an insufficient ethical framework for promoting ethical deci-sion making with families in the context of cultural differences. Cultural variability in interpretation of what constitutes harm may make discussions based on the principle of nonmaleficence diffi-cult. Similarly, cultural variation in the interpretation of autonomy may lead to different perceptions of its value in informed consent as some cultures view autonomy to reflect the need to respect the pa-tient, but not directly tied to decision making.[60]

Others have criticized the principle-based approach as overly narrow, instead recognizing that complex health care decision making is deeply contextual and rooted in intertwined relationships between family and society, children and parents, and other family members. Narrative ethics frameworks that recognize the interests of patients as relationally embedded in the interests of others have been proposed as an alternative.[60-63] Cultural humility under these theories requires relational ethics inquiry, incorporating patient narratives to understand the principles and metaphors expressed by patients and families that reflect their cultural diversity.

Finally, cultural humility requires that the moral relevance of mi-nority viewpoints is not overlooked by those in the majority.

Conclusion and Recommendations

The multidimensional, dynamic nature of culture, and the well-documented connection between patient-provider cul-tural differences and health outcomes, makes it imperative that providers, hospitals, and health care systems adopt a stance of cul-tural humility, built on the same principles that underlie patient-and family-centered care.[64] This is especially important in the context of complex decision making when many facets of an individual's culture may impact their values and preferences, their communication styles, their relationship to clinicians, and their interactions with the health care system.

The following recommendations may help providers ensure high-quality communication and SDM for all patients, regardless of cultural background.

Avoid self-referentialism.[37] Whether or not we share the same race, religion, socioeconomic, educational, or geographic background as our patients and families, health care providers are always inherently operating within a cross-cultural dynamic due to the culture that medicine bears within itself, which is associated with its own language, values, and worldview. Feminist standpoint theory reminds us that we are all "situated knowers," that is, what we believe we know is dependent on our social location and individual experiences.[65] If we assume that our understanding (of a particular situation, of ethical norms, or of the world in general) is the only correct one, we will find ourselves in conflict with others on a regular basis.

Beware of homogenization. It is easy to take what is known about a patient or family and create a narrative that is then used to understand, explain, and predict their behavior. This singular story ignores the multiple, heterogeneous truths that dictate all life experiences and does not honor the complexity of human existence. Approaching families and patients with attention to their human dignity and interest in the complexity of their story builds trust and allows more complete understanding that will reduce communication breakdown along cultural lines.[66]

Practice cultural humility. The concept of cultural humility goes beyond cultural competence to incorporate lifelong learning, inquisitiveness, and self-reflection and critique.[67] It is especially important in the context of medical decision making, where power imbalances are always present. Cultural humility reminds us to ask questions and listen with openness that helps us avoid the traps of cultural stereotypes and assumptions. Cultural humility also reminds us of the fluid nature of culture and the importance of revisiting the values, beliefs, and behaviors of patients and families whose cultural influences may shift during the experience of caring for a sick loved one.

Cultivate self-awareness. An element of the art of medicine lies in a consciousness of the cultural biases we carry as health care providers and the ability to transcend the differences between ourselves and our patients by finding points of human connection. Engaging our skills in empathy—the willingness to be present with our patients, to listen, and to genuinely attempt to understand what they are feeling—is a key component of this process.

Respect patient/family preferences for SDM. Individual patients and families will have different preferences for their level of involvement in decision making, as well as the preferred degree of provider participation. Some will prefer high levels of patient/family-directed decision making, while others will prefer a high level of provider involvement and/or direction in decision making. Both perspectives are likely to be deeply influenced by culture. The most effective providers will be able to shift their level of involvement in decision making based on patient and family needs.[1,68]

Acknowledge the moral relevance of culture. The essence of culture involves powerful and defining moral experiences that are at the very core of one's identity.[5] An individual's cultural connection to their social structures and community is essential to coping with a significant health care experience. For most pediatric patients, this connection is primarily accomplished in and through their family. Failure to acknowledge culture as an important aspect of moral experience (for providers as well as patients and families) risks underappreciating the foundation of SDM in informed consent and respect for persons. Conversely, taking the time to understand the culture, values, and beliefs of patients and families will help providers to support the family in an SDM process that leads to well-informed and authentic decisions.

The knowledge and skills to provide culturally effective health care can be taught to health care providers and students. However, without attention to workforce diversity and the broader context of health disparities, the impact of this education will be limited. Addressing the educational and organizational barriers that prevent meaningful diversity within the health care workforce is a crucial component of advocacy work.[69]

The data reviewed for this chapter represents a sampling of current literature on the subject. Many unanswered questions remain that will require collaborative work between specialists in communication and decision-making research, health literacy, social determinants of health, and health policy, among others.[70] This multidisciplinary research must be grounded in patient- and family-centered outcomes and open to redirection from community participants to achieve meaningful results.

In the coming years, we are hopeful to see continued improvement in the authenticity of cross-cultural interactions and the quality of SDM in medicine. The growing emphasis on SDM as standard of care and shifting demographics in the age of globalization will help spur this change. Because of the commitment to advocacy and family-centered care that is so central to pediatrics, pediatric health care providers are well situated to lead this critically important effort.

References

1. Kon AA. Difficulties in judging patient preferences for shared decision-making. *J Med Ethics*. 2012;38(12):719–720.
2. Azoulay E, Pochard F, Chevret S, et al. Half the family members of intensive care unit patients do not want to share in the decision-making process: a study in 78 French intensive care units. *Crit Care Med*. 2004;32(9):1832–1838.
3. Cochran D, Saleem S, Khowaja-Punjwani S, Lantos JD. Cross-cultural differences in communication about a dying child. *Pediatrics*. 2017;140(5):e20170690.

4. Crenshaw K, Shewchuk RM, Qu H, et al. What should we include in a cultural competence curriculum? An emerging formative evaluation process to foster curriculum development. *Acad Med.* 2011;86(3):333–341.

5. Kleinman A, Benson P. Culture, moral experience and medicine. *Mt Sinai J Med.* 2006;73(6):834–839.

6. Seeleman C, Suurmond J, Stronks K. Cultural competence: a conceptual framework for teaching and learning. *Med Educ.* 2009;43(3):229–237.

7. Perkins HS. Culture as a useful conceptual tool in clinical ethics consultation. *Camb Q Healthc Ethics.* 2008;17(2):164–172.

8. Aviv R. What does it mean to die? *New Yorker.* February 5, 2018.

9. Derrington SF, Paquette E, Johnson KA. Cross-cultural interactions and shared decision-making. *Pediatrics.* 2018;142(Suppl 3):S187–S192.

10. Richardson A, Allen JA, Xiao H, Vallone D. Effects of race/ethnicity and socioeconomic status on health information-seeking, confidence, and trust. *J Health Care Poor Underserved.* 2012;23(4):1477–1493.

11. Lee JJ, Long AC, Curtis JR, Engelberg RA. The influence of race/ethnicity and education on family ratings of the quality of dying in the ICU. *J Pain Symptom Manage.* 2016;51(1):9–16.

12. Harris VC, Links AR, Walsh J, et al. A systematic review of race/ethnicity and parental treatment decision-making. *Clin Pediatr.* 2018;57(12):1453–1464.

13. Michelson KN, Patel R, Haber-Baker N, Emanuel L, Frader J. End of life care decisions in the pediatric intensive care unit: roles professionals play. *Pediatr Crit Care.* 2013;14(1):34–44.

14. Madrigal V, Carroll KW, Faerber JA, Walter JK, Morrison WE, Feudtner C. Parental sources of guidance when making difficult decisions in the pediatric intensive care unit. *J Pediatri.* 2016;169:221–226.

15. Arutyunyan T, Odetola F, Swieringa R, Niedner M. Religion and spiritual care in pediatric intensive care unit: parental attitudes regarding physician spiritual and religious inquiry. *Am J Hosp Palliat Care.* 2018;35(1):28–33.

16. Catlin EA, Cadge W, Ecklund EH, Gage EA, Zollfrank AA. The spiritual and religious identities, beliefs, and practices of academic pediatricians in the United States. *Acad Med.* 2008;83(12):1146–1152.

17. Ecklund EH, Cadge W, Gage EA, Catlin EA. The religious and spiritual beliefs and practices of academic pediatric oncologists in the United States. *J Pediatr Hematol Oncol.* 2007;29(11):736–742.

18. Bowman M, St Cyr S, Stolf IA. Health-care provider personal religious preferences and their perspectives on advance care planning with patients. *Am J Hosp Palliat Care.* 2018;35(12):1565–1571.

19. Hexem KR, Mollen CJ, Carroll K, Lanctot DA, Feudtner C. How parents of children receiving pediatric palliative care use religion, spirituality, or life philosophy in tough times. *J Palliat Med.* 2011;14(1):39–44.

20. Superdock AK, Barfield RC, Brandon DH, Docherty SL. Exploring the vagueness of religion and spirituality in complex pediatric decision-making: a qualitative study. *BMC Palliat Care*. 2018;17(1):107.

21. Druml C, Ballmer PE, Druml W, et al. ESPEN guideline on ethical aspects of artificial nutrition and hydration. *Clin Nutr*. 2016;35(3):545–556.

22. Alsolamy S. Islamic views on artificial nutrition and hydration in terminally ill patients. *Bioethics*. 2014;28(2):96–99.

23. Drane JF. Stopping nutrition and hydration technologies: a conflict between traditional Catholic ethics and church authority. *Christ Bioeth*. 2006;12(1):11–28.

24. Wiener L, McConnell DG, Latella L, Ludi E. Cultural and religious considerations in pediatric palliative care. *Palliat Support Care*. 2013;11(1):47–67.

25. Tay K, Yu Lee RJ, Sim SW, Menon S, Kanesvaran R, Radha Krishna LK. Cultural influences upon advance care planning in a family-centric society. *Palliat Support Care*. 2017;15(6):665–674.

26. Gordon M. Rituals in death and dying: modern medical technologies enter the fray. *Rambam Maimonides Med J*. 2015;6(1):e0007.

27. Bosslet GT, Pope TM, Rubenfeld GD, et al. An official ATS/AACN/ACCP/ESICM/SCCM policy statement: responding to requests for potentially inappropriate treatments in intensive care units. *Am J Respir Crit Care Med*. 2015;191(11):1318–1330.

28. Schweda M, Schicktanz S, Raz A, Silvers A. Beyond cultural stereotyping: views on end-of-life decision making among religious and secular persons in the USA, Germany, and Israel. *BMC Med Ethics*. 2017;18(1):13.

29. Kon AA. Informed non-dissent: a better option than slow codes when families cannot bear to say "let her die." *Am J Bioeth*. 2011;11(11):22–23.

30. Hinds PS, Oakes LL, Hicks J, et al. "Trying to be a good parent" as defined by interviews with parents who made phase I, terminal care, and resuscitation decisions for their children. *J Clin Oncol*. 2009;27(35):5979–5985.

31. Bluebond-Langner M. *The Private Worlds of Dying Children*. Princeton, NJ: Princeton University Press; 1978.

32. Skrzypek M. The social origin of the illness experience—an outline of problems. *Ann Agric Environ Med*. 2014;21(3):654–660.

33. Conrad P, Barker KK. The social construction of illness: key insights and policy implications. *J Health Soc Behav*. 2010;(51 Suppl):S67–S79.

34. Rosenberg AR, Starks H, Unguru Y, Feudtner C, Diekema D. Truth telling in the setting of cultural differences and incurable pediatric illness: a review. *JAMA Pediatr*. 2017;171(11):1113–1119.

35. Foster MJ, Whitehead L, Maybee P, Cullens V. The parents', hospitalized child's, and health care providers' perceptions and experiences of family

centered care within a pediatric critical care setting: a metasynthesis of qualitative research. *J Fam Nurs.* 2013;19(4):431–468.

36. Marcus KL, Henderson CM, Boss RD. Chronic critical illness in infants and children: a speculative synthesis on adapting ICU care to meet the needs of long-stay patients. *Pediatr Crit Care Med.* 2016;17(8):743–752.

37. Brannigan MC. Connecting the dots in cultural competency: institutional strategies and conceptual caveats. *Camb Q Healthc Ethics.* 2008;17:173–184.

38. Oberle K, Hughes D. Doctors' and nurses' perspectives of ethical problems in end-of-life decisions. *J Adv Nurs.* 2001;33(6):707–715.

39. Hamric AB, Blackhall LJ. Nurse-physician perspectives on the care of dying patients in intensive care units: collaboration, moral distress, and ethical climate. *Crit Care Med.* 2007;35:422–429.

40. McAndrew NS. Nurses and physicians bring different perspectives to end-of-life decisions in intensive care units. *Evid-Based Nurs.* 2018;21(3):85. doi:10.1136/eb-2018-102902.

41. Balkin EM, Sleeper LA, Kirkpatrick JN, et al. Physician perspectives on palliative care for children with advanced heart disease: a comparison between pediatric cardiology and palliative care physicians. *J Palliat Med.* 2018;21(6):774–779.

42. Ciriello AG, Dizon ZB, October TW. Speaking a different language: a qualitative analysis comparing language of palliative care and pediatric intensive care unit physicians. *Am J Hosp Palliat Med.* 2018;35(3):384–389.

43. Iannello P, Perucca V, Riva S, Antonietti A, Pravettoni G. What do physicians believe about the way decisions are made? A pilot study on metacognitive knowledge in the medical context. *Eur J Psychol.* 2015;11(4):691–706.

44. Maina IW, Belton TD, Ginzberg S, Singh A, Johnson TJ. A decade of studying implicit racial/ethnic bias in healthcare providers using the implicit association test. *Soc Sci Med.* 2018;199:219–229.

45. McGary H. Racial groups, distrust, and the distribution of health care. In: Rhodes R, Battin MP, Silvers A, eds. *Medicine and Social Justice: Essays on the Distribution of Health Care.* New York: Oxford University Press; 2012:265–278.

46. Periyakoil VS, Neri E, Kramer H. No easy talk: a mixed methods study of doctor reported barriers to conducting effective end-of-life conversations with diverse patients. *PloS One.* 2015;10(4):e0122321.

47. Talati ED, Lang CW, Ross LF. Reactions of pediatricians to refusals of medical treatment for minors. *J Adolesc Health.* 2010;47(2):126–132.

48. Committee on B. Conflicts between religious or spiritual beliefs and pediatric care: informed refusal, exemptions, and public funding. *Pediatrics.* 2013;132(5):962–965.

49. Brierley J, Linthicum J, Petros A. Should religious beliefs be allowed to stonewall a secular approach to withdrawing and withholding treatment in children? *J Med Ethics*. 2013;39(9):573–577.

50. Seale C. The role of doctors' religious faith and ethnicity in taking ethically controversial decisions during end-of-life care. *J Med Ethics*. 2010;36(11):677–682.

51. Sharma RK, Dy SM. Cross-cultural communication and use of the family meeting in palliative care. *Am J Hosp Palliat Care*. 2011;28(6):437–444.

52. Diekema DS. Parental refusals of medical treatment: the harm principle as threshold for state intervention. *Theor Med Bioeth*. 2004;25(4):243–264.

53. Hagiwara N, Penner LA, Gonzalez R, et al. Racial attitudes, physician-patient talk time ratio, and adherence in racially discordant interactions. *Soc Sci Med*. 2013;87:123–131.

54. Elliott AM, Alexander SC, Mescher CA, Mohan D, Barnato AE. Differences in physicians' verbal and nonverbal communication with black and white patients at the end of life. *J Pain Symptom Manage*. 2016;51(1):1–8.

55. Mack JW, Paulk E, Viswanath K, Prigerson HG. Racial disparities in the outcomes of communication on medical care received near death. *Arch Intern Med*. 2010;170(17):1533–1540.

56. Anand KJ, Sepanski RJ, Giles K, Shah SH, Juarez PD. Pediatric intensive care unit mortality among Latino children before and after a multilevel health care delivery intervention. *JAMA Pediatr*. 2015;169(4):383–390.

57. McKee MM, Paasche-Orlow MK. Health literacy and the disenfranchised: the importance of collaboration between limited English proficiency and health literacy researchers. *J Health Commun*. 2012;17(Suppl 3):7–12.

58. Hayes B, Fabri AM, Coperchini M, Parkar R, Austin-Crowe Z. Health and death literacy and cultural diversity: insights from hospital-employed interpreters. *BMJ Support Palliat Care*. 2020;10(1):e8.

59. Gengler AM. "I want you to save my kid!": illness management strategies, access, and inequality at an elite university research hospital. *J Health Soc Behav*. 2014;55(3):342–359.

60. Westra AE, Willems DL, Smit BJ. Communicating with Muslim parents: "the four principles" are not as culturally neutral as suggested. *J Pediatr*. 2009;168(11):1383–1387.

61. Carnevale FAP, Teachman G, Bogossian A. A relational ethics framework for advancing practice with children with complex health care needs and their parents. *Compr Child Adolesc Nurs*. 2017;40(4):268–284.

62. Pesut B. Incorporating patients' spirituality into care using Gadow's ethical framework. *Nurs Ethics*. 2009;16(4):418–428.

63. Johnstone MJ. Bioethics, cultural differences, and the problem of moral disagreements in end-of-life care: a terror management theory. *J Med Philos*. 2012;37(2):181–200.

64. Epner DE, Baile WF. Patient-centered care: the key to cultural competence. *Ann Oncol.* 2012;23(Suppl 3):33–42.
65. Grasswick H. Feminist social epistemology. In: Zalta EN, ed. *The Stanford Encyclopedia of Philosophy.* 2016.
66. Adiche C. The danger of a single story. *TED Talks.* 2009.
67. Fahlberg B, Foronda C, Baptiste D. Cultural humility: the key to patient/family partnerships for making difficult decisions. *Nursing.* 2016;46(9):14–16.
68. Curtis JR, White DB. Practical guidance for evidence-based ICU family conferences. *Chest.* 2008;134(4):835–843.
69. American Academy of Pediatrics Committee on Pediatric Workforce. Enhancing pediatric workforce diversity and providing culturally effective pediatric care: implications for practice, education, and policy making. *Pediatrics.* 2013;132(4):e1105–e16.
70. Tulsky JA, Beach MC, Butow PN, et al. A research agenda for communication between health care professionals and patients living with serious illness. *JAMA Intern Med.* 2017;177(9):1361–1366.

11

Biases and Heuristics That Subtly Shape Decisions

Jennifer Blumenthal-Barby

Biases and Heuristics in Decision Making: A Brief Overview

Decision scientists have demonstrated that people often use decision-making shortcuts ("heuristics") that can lead to predictable biases in judgment and decision making. For example, we are more influenced by what we hear first and last in a stream of information. Information framed in terms of loss (e.g., mortality percentage) is more influential than the same information framed in terms of gain (e.g., survival percentage). We feel more at risk when we receive risk information in relative terms (e.g., fivefold increase) than absolute terms (e.g., 1% to 5%) and in terms of frequencies (e.g., 2 in 10) than percentages (e.g., 20%). We tend to go with whatever is presented as the default, and we are especially averse to "doing" something to cause harm—even if not doing something causes more harm. We can fall prey to sunk costs whereby we continue to do something we are not benefiting from just because we already invested time or money into it. We are strongly influenced by the power of social norms and what others do or choose, especially if those people are perceived as similar to us or as authority figures. We underestimate our ability to adapt to negative events and overestimate the chance that good outcomes will happen to us compared to other people. And the list goes on.

These psychological tendencies have been named, studied, and validated by behavioral economists and decision scientists over the past several decades. Table 11.1 provides a summary of some of the most well-studied heuristics and biases that have been shown to play a role in medical decision making.

Impact on Patient Decision Making and Philosophical Implications

Impact on Patient Decision Making

How have these heuristics and biases (henceforth, H&Bs) been shown to impact patients' medical decision making? In a systematic review of studies of H&Bs in medical decision making, my colleague and I found a total of 140 studies that assessed H&Bs in patients' decision making, and 61% confirmed the presence of the heuristic or bias investigated.[19]

The most well-studied and confirmed biases included the loss/gain framing bias, the relative risk bias, and the availability bias. Others included omission bias, primacy and recency biases, impact bias, optimism bias, and bandwagon effect.

In one study of the loss/gain framing bias, researchers found that significantly more patients would consent to angioplasty when told that "99 in 100 have no complications" (gain frame) than when told that "1 in 100 have complications" (loss frame).[20] In a study of the relative risk bias, researchers found that participants receiving information about relative risk reduction were 3.1 to 5.8 times more likely to take statins than those receiving information framed in terms of absolute risk reduction, number needed to treat, event rates, tablets needed to take, and natural frequencies (whole numbers).[21] In a study of the availability bias, researchers found that women's decision making regarding whether to delay or seek diagnosis of breast cancer depended in part on how easily they could

Table 11.1. Types of Biases and Heuristics Empirically Studied in Medical Decision Making

Bias/Heuristic	Definition
Affect Heuristic	"Representations of objects and events in people's minds are tagged to varying degrees with affect. People consult or refer to an 'affective pool' (containing all the positive and negative tags associated with the representations consciously or unconsciously) in the process of making judgments"[1]
Ambiguity Aversion	The display of preferences for known or certain probabilities over uncertain probabilities regardless of actual benefits[2]
Anchoring Bias	"The response is strongly biased toward any value, even if it is arbitrary, that the respondent is induced to consider as a candidate answer"[3]
Availability Bias	"People assess the frequency of a class or the probability of an event by the ease with which instances or occurrences can be brought to mind"[4]
Bandwagon Effect	"An accelerating diffusion through a group or population of a pattern of behaviour, the probability of any individual adopting it increasing with the proportion who have already done so"[5]
Commission Bias	"Tendency toward action rather than inaction"[6]
Confirmation Bias	"The tendency to perceive more support for [one's] beliefs than actually exists in the evidence at hand"[7]
Decoy Effect	"The addition of such [asymmetrically dominated] alternatives increases the share of the item that dominates it"[8]
Default Bias or Status Quo Bias	"Individuals have a strong tendency to remain at the status quo, because the disadvantages of leaving it loom larger than advantages"[9]
Frequency/ Percentage Framing Effect	"Frequency scales generally . . . lead to higher perceived risk"[10]
Impact Bias	"Failure to anticipate our remarkable ability to adapt to new states. People tend to overestimate the long-term impact of both positive events . . . and negative events"[11]

Continued

Table 11.1. Continued

Bias/Heuristic	Definition
Loss/Gain Framing Bias or Loss Aversion Bias	"Losses loom larger than corresponding gains"[12]
Omission Bias	"Judge harmful commissions as worse than the corresponding omissions"[13]
Optimism Bias or Optimistic Overconfidence	"Tendency to undervalue those aspects of the situation of which the judge is relatively ignorant . . . [and have] favorable expectations for [an] activity, and for their own prospects in particular"[14]
Order Effects: Primacy/ Recency	Information presented at the beginning or end of a series is remembered and chosen more often than information presented in the middle of the series[15] (p. 569)
Outcome Bias	Allowing a prior event or decision outcome to influence subsequent independent decisions[16]
Relative Risk Bias	"A stronger inclination to [choose treatment] when presented with the relative . . . risk than when presented with the same [information] described in terms of the absolute . . . risk"[17]
Representativeness Heuristic	"Probabilities are evaluated by the degree to which A is representative of B, that is, by the degree to which A resembles B . . . [and] not influenced by factors that should affect judgments . . . prior probability outcomes . . . sample size . . . chance . . . predictability . . . validity"[14]
Sunk Cost Effect	"Tendency to continue an endeavor once an investment in money, effort, or time has been made"[18]

Originally published in Blumenthal-Barby and Krieger 2015.

recall stories of women who sought early diagnosis with a good outcome (for diagnosis seekers) or women who had bad outcomes (for diagnosis delayers).[22]

An example of the impact of the omission bias on patients' decision making can be seen in a study of vaccination decision making. Researchers found that parents who did not or would now allow their child to be vaccinated against pertussis were more likely to favor potentially harmful omissions over less harmful acts.[23] Primacy and recency biases have been shown to impact patient decision making in a variety of contexts. One example of the recency bias involves the finding that women who learned about the risks of tamoxifen first (for breast cancer prevention) thought more favorably of the drug than women who learned about the benefits first.[24] In a display of the impact bias, healthy participants failed to anticipate their ability to adapt to negative events and rated the happiness of dialysis patients as much lower than that actually reported by dialysis patients (in fact, their actual well-being nearly matched that of healthy controls).[25] Optimism bias was on display in patients with renal failure who overestimated the impact of a transplant on various domains of quality of life (e.g., travel, work, energy).[26] And finally, bandwagon effect has been found to impact patients' decision making in several types of vaccination contexts. One study found that social norms were a dominant determinant of college women's decision making about the human papillomavirus vaccine.[27]

Philosophical and Ethical Implications

These findings regarding how patients use H&Bs to arrive at decisions have implications for how we think about the normative dimensions of decision making by and with patients. Clearly, H&Bs shape people's understanding of their options and the likely consequences of those options. Moreover, they shape the extent to which patients' decisions are intentional and deliberative versus intuitive and reflexive. Finally, they can shape the extent to which patients' choices reflect their underlying values. In all of these ways, H&Bs influence patient autonomy, since understanding, intentionality, and values-based decision making are key components of truly autonomous choice.[28]

There are some ways in which H&Bs can *enhance* autonomous choice. For example, one might argue that increased response to loss-framed information can be thought of as a patient coming to understand and appreciate risk in a much deeper way than they had previously. A patient who hears the situation as "99 in 100 have no complications" might dismiss or fail to give due consideration to the possibility that they might be the unlucky one who has complications, and only seriously consider this when they hear the "1 in 100 have complications" frame.

In most cases, however, H&Bs are likely to *threaten* autonomous choice rather than enhance it, at least based on how autonomy has traditionally been understood in bioethics. For example, if a patient feels "really at risk," when the odds of complication are just 1 in 100, then they misunderstand (either affectively and/or cognitively). In a different example, if, due to an optimism bias, a transplant candidate overestimates the number of days they will be able to work or overestimates their overall quality of life, then they misunderstand these matters. If, due to an impact bias, a patient considering dialysis believes that life with dialysis is much more negative than it actually is, they misunderstand in a significant way. This is all on the understanding front. Intentional and deliberate decision making can also be negatively impacted by H&Bs. H&Bs often operate by *bypassing* deliberative and intentional decision making.

Finally, H&Bs can threaten the extent to which patients' choices match their underlying values. Consider a patient who, due to a bandwagon effect, decides to "do whatever other people do." It is not the *patient's* values driving their choice, but the values and preferences of others. Or, consider a patient who chooses an option (e.g., life-sustaining treatment on an advance directive) simply because it is presented as the default—it is not their values that determine the choice, but the framing of the form.[29]

Consider a patient who had always valued quality of life over quantity of life, but who finds themselves pressing for more treatment in the intensive care unit because of the sunk cost effect ("We've gone this far down the road . . .").

One way to put the threat to autonomy is to employ a distinction drawn by Dan Brudney and John Lantos between two elements of autonomy: agency and authenticity. Agency refers to the capacity choose, to take something as a "sufficient reason" to act (as opposed to merely responding to desires and whims as they occur).[30] Authenticity, on the other hand, refers to "living one's own distinctive life, to constructing one's life in accordance with one's distinctive beliefs and values." Authentic choices reflect who the patient is, their character, life narrative, and values. Authenticity refers not just to our capacity to decide and to act, but to our capacity to do so in a way that reflects *our* values. Perhaps the component of autonomy that H&Bs threaten most is authenticity (though there is certainly an argument to be made that agency is threatened as well).

All of this opens up the possibility that clinicians need to do more than simply deliver information and elicit values from patients during decision making in order to respect and promote autonomy. They need to understand patients' H&Bs and frame choices in a way that increases the likelihood that their choices will reflect their values. I will discuss this possibility (sometimes called "choice architecture" or "nudging" of patient decision making) more in the next section, but before doing so we must also consider how H&Bs impact clinicians' decision making.

Impact on Clinician Decision Making and Philosophical Implications

Impact on Clinician Decision Making

Clinicians are equally susceptible to H&Bs in their decision making. Our 2015 review of the literature found a total of 64 studies that assessed H&Bs in the decision making of medical personnel (i.e., an individual with at least some medical training making a decision regarding diagnosis, prognosis, treatment, or assessment of another individual's care). Eighty percent of studies confirmed the presence of the heuristic or bias assessed. In an example of loss/gain framing bias, physicians projected better survival from lung cancer when asked to predict the chance of patients "dying within" (e.g., 6 months) rather than "living at least" (e.g., 6 months).[31] Clinicians are also susceptible to the relative risk bias. Physicians were asked how willing they would be to prescribe certain drugs when learning of clinical trial results. Researchers found that in the relative risk reduction frame, 77% were likely to prescribe the drug, compared to 24% in the absolute risk reduction frame, 37% in the event-free patients frame, and 34% in the number needed to treat frame.[32] The impact of availability bias on clinician decision making can be seen in a study of physicians' prescribing behavior. Physicians who had a recent patient with an adverse bleeding event from warfarin were 21% less likely to prescribe the drug to other patients for 90 days after.[33]

Omission bias has also been shown to impact clinician decision making. For example, one study found that pulmonologists were more likely to choose a suboptimal management option (against guidelines) for the evaluation of pulmonary embolism and for the treatment of septic shock when an omission option (do nothing/preserve status quo chain of events) was given to them.[34] Primacy and recency biases (order effects) are also a factor. Researchers found that physicians who heard a patient's history and physical information last (*after* lab data) were more likely to diagnose the patient with a urinary tract infection (UTI) (the H&P were suggestive of UTI; the lab data was not) compared with physicians who received the reverse ordering.[35]

Impact bias occurs when people fail to anticipate the human ability to adapt and overestimate the long-term impact of negative and positive events. Clinicians may fail to adequately anticipate patients' abilities to adapt to negative health events/states and, as a result, overestimate how bad some negative event might feel to patients actually undergoing that event or health state. For example, one study found that clinicians' attitudes toward chemotherapy were much more negative than patients'.[36] Various factors likely explain this difference, but one might be failure to recognize the power of adaptation. This is often the case when "able-bodied" persons consider what life might be like for persons with a "disability" (who are differently abled). Finally, optimism biases and frequency biases can also impact clinicians' decision making. One study found that physicians overestimated the survival time of patients referred to hospice by a factor of 5.3.[37] Frequency bias was demonstrated by a study that found that 41% of psychiatrists said they would refuse to discharge a patient whose risk of violence was 20 in 100, whereas only 21% who received the percentage frame (20%) said they would refuse to discharge such a patient.[38]

Philosophical and Ethical Implications

Earlier, I argued that H&Bs can shape patient autonomy and that clinicians ought to recognize this and engage in choice architecture that considers how H&Bs work with the aim of enhancing patient understanding (cognitive and affective) and increasing the likelihood that the patient's choice reflects their values. For example, if a clinician senses that a patient is feeling very at risk about an angioplasty due to having heard that 1 in 100 have complications, they can inform the patient that that also means that 99 in 100 do not have complications. If a patient is delaying seeking a breast cancer diagnosis due to an availability bias triggered by stories of women who had sought early diagnosis and had bad outcomes, the clinician might remind the patient of stories of women who had delayed diagnosis and had bad outcomes—and who had sought early diagnosis and had good outcomes. If a patient is refusing a vaccination due to an omission bias, the clinician can frame not vaccinating as an act as well (one that is more harmful). If a patient values minimizing medical intervention and is facing a localized, early-stage prostate cancer diagnosis, the clinician can normalize the choice of active surveillance by informing the patient that many other men do choose that option.

There is, however, a paradox here: if clinicians themselves are susceptible to H&Bs, how can they improve patient choice? How can they see their way through their own H&Bs to help a patient understand in the way that they need to, or to help them make a choice that truly reflects their values (as opposed to reflecting the clinicians' own biases)? For example, perhaps the clinician discussing angioplasty just had a case where their patient *did* have some of those rare complications and, as a result, under the influence of availability bias, nudges the patient away from it by emphasizing the risk (1 in 100 have complications). Perhaps a clinician treating a patient in the intensive care unit is also under the influence of sunk cost. Perhaps a clinician treating a patient with chemotherapy underestimates how much a patient values the additional weeks or months of life.

In these cases, H&Bs put clinicians at risk for getting both the medical facts wrong (or distorted) and the patients' values wrong. There is no easy remedy to this. One implication is the need for epistemic humility. There are practical steps that can be taken in light of such humility—for example, checking oneself for known H&Bs, enlisting help from colleagues to check judgment and decision making, taking time and care to elicit rather than assume patient values, etc. Clinicians are arguably in a better position than patients to hone their skills in dealing with H&Bs in medical decision making since they make medical decisions day in and day out, and most patients only make such decisions as "one off" or here and there.

Conclusion

In sum, empirical research on the psychology of decision making, including research into decisional H&Bs, is of great importance for the study and practice of decision making by patients, by clinicians, and between patients and clinicians. This research shows that decisions are made and shaped in ways far more subtle than has traditionally been appreciated. As such, it presents nuances and challenges for our thinking about core bioethics concepts such as autonomy, informed consent, and shared decision making.

References

1. Isen AM, Rosenzweig AS, Young MJ. The influence of positive affect on clinical problem solving. *Med Decis Mak.* 1991;11(3):221–227.
2. Fox CR, Tversky A. Ambiguity aversion and comparative ignorance. In: Kahneman D, Tversky A, eds. *Choices, Values, and Frames.* New York: Russell Sage Foundation, Cambridge University Press; 2000:528–542.
3. Kahneman D, Knetsch JL, Thaler RH. Anomalies: the endowment effect, loss aversion, and status quo bias. In: Kahneman D, Tversky A, eds. *Choices, Values, and Frames.* New York: Russell Sage Foundation, Cambridge University Press; 2000:159–170.
4. Kahneman D, Tversky A. Introduction judgment under uncertainty: heuristics and biases. In: Kahneman D, Slovic P, Tversky A, eds. *Judgment Under Uncertainty: Heuristics and Biases.* New York: Cambridge University Press; 1982.
5. Colman A. Group think: bandwagon effect. In: *Oxford Dictionary of Psychology.* New York: Oxford University Press; 2003:77.
6. Croskerry P. Achieving quality in clinical decision making: cognitive strategies and detection of bias. *Acad Emerg Med.* 2002;9(11):1184–1204.
7. Ross L, Anderson CA. Shortcomings in the attribution process: on the origins and maintenance of erroneous social assessments. In: Kahneman D, Slovic P, Tversky A, eds. *Judgment Under Uncertainty: Heuristics and Biases.* New York: Cambridge University Press; 1982.
8. Huber J, Payne JW, Puto C. Adding asymmetrically dominated alternatives: violations of regularity and the similarity hypothesis. *J Consum Res.* 1982;9(1):90–98.
9. Kahneman D, Ritov I, Schkade D. Economic preferences or attitude expression? An analysis of dollar responses to public issues. In: Kahneman D, Tversky A, eds. *Choices, Values, and Frames.* New York: Russell Sage Foundation, Cambridge University Press; 2000:642–672.
10. Slovic P, Monahan J, MacGregor DG. Violence risk assessment and risk communication: the effects of using actual cases, providing instruction, and employing probability versus frequency formats. *Law Hum Behav.* 2000;24(3):271–296.

11. Griffin D, Tversky A. Endowments and contrast in judgments of well-being. In: Kahneman D, Tversky A, eds. *Choices, Values, and Frames.* New York: Russell Sage Foundation, Cambridge University Press; 2000:709–725.

12. Kahneman D, Thaler RH, Knetsch J. Loss aversion in riskless choice: a reference-dependent model. In: Kahneman D, Tversky A, eds. *Choices, Values, and Frames.* New York: Russell Sage Foundation, Cambridge University Press; 2000:143–158.

13. Spranca M, Minsk E, Baron J. Omission and commission in judgment and choice. *J Exper Soc Psychol.* 1991;27(1):76–105.

14. Kahneman D, Tversky A. Conflict resolution: a cognitive perspective. In: Kahneman D, Tversky A, eds. *Choices, Values, and Frames.* New York: Russell Sage Foundation, Cambridge University Press; 2000:473–488.

15. Loewenstein G, Prelec D. Preferences for sequences of outcomes. In: Kahneman D, Tversky A, eds. *Choices, Values, and Frames.* New York: Russell Sage Foundation, Cambridge University Press; 2000:565–596.

16. Einhorn HJ. Learning from experience and suboptimal rules in decision making. In: Kahneman D, Slovic P, Tversky A, eds. *Judgment Under Uncertainty: Heuristics and Biases.* New York: Cambridge University Press; 1982:1082–1092.

17. Forrow L, Taylor WC, Arnold RM. Absolutely relative: how research results are summarized can affect treatment decisions. *Am J Med.* 1992;92(2):121–124.

18. Arkes HR, Blumer C. The psychology of sunk cost. *Organ Behav Hum Decis Process.* 1985;35(1):124–140.

19. Blumenthal-Barby JS, Krieger H. Cognitive biases and heuristics in medical decision making: a critical review using a systematic search strategy. *Med Decis Mak.* 2015;35(4):539–557.

20. Gurm HS, Litaker DG. Framing procedural risks to patients:is 99% safe the same as a risk of 1 in 100? *Acad Med.* 2000;75(8):840–842.

21. Carling C, Kristoffersen DT, Herrin J, et al. How should the impact of different presentations of treatment effects on patient choice be evaluated? A pilot randomized trial. *PloS One.* 2008;3(11):e3693. https://doi.org/10.1371/journal.pone.0003693.

22. Facione NC, Facione PA. The cognitive structuring of patient delay in breast cancer. *Soc Sci Med.* 2006;63(12):3137–3149. https://doi.org/10.1016/j.socscimed.2006.08.014.

23. Asch DA, Baron J, Hershey JC, et al. Omission bias and pertussis vaccination. *Med Decis Mak.* 1994;14(2):118–123. https://doi.org/10.1177/0272989X9401400204.

24. Ubel PA, Smith DM, Zikmund-Fisher BJ, et al. Testing whether decision aids introduce cognitive biases: results of a randomized trial. *Patient Educ Couns.* 2010;80(2):158–163. https://doi.org/10.1016/j.pec.2009.10.021.

25. Riis J, Loewenstein G, Baron J, Jepson C, Fagerlin A, Ubel PA. Ignorance of hedonic adaptation to hemodialysis: a study using ecological momentary assessment. *J Exper Psychol: Gen.* 2005;134(1):3–9. https://doi.org/10.1037/0096-3445.134.1.3.

26. Smith D, Loewenstein G, Jepson C, Jankovich A, Feldman H, Ubel P. Mispredicting and misremembering: patients with renal failure overestimate improvements in quality of life after a kidney transplant. *Health Psychol.* 2008;27(5):653–658. https://doi.org/10.1037/a0012647.

27. Allen JD, Mohllajee AP, Shelton RC, Othus MKD, Fontenot HB, Hanna R. Stage of adoption of the human papillomavirus vaccine among college women. *Prevent Med.* 2009;48(5):420–425. https://doi.org/10.1016/j.ypmed.2008.12.005.

28. Faden RR, Beauchamp TL. *A History and Theory of Informed Consent.* New York: Oxford University Press; 1986

29. Halpern SD, Loewenstein G, Volpp KG, et al. Default options in advance directives influence how patients set goals for end-of-life care. *Health Aff.* 2013;32(2):408–417.

30. Brudney D, Lantos J. Agency and authenticity: which value grounds patient choice? *Theor Med Bioeth.* 2011;32(4):217–227.

31. Quartin AA, Calonge RO, Schein RMH, Crandall LA. Influence of critical illness on physicians' prognoses for underlying disease: a randomized study using simulated cases. *Crit Care Med.* 2008;36(2):462–470.

32. Bobbio M, Demichelis B, Giustetto G. Completeness of reporting trial results: effect on physicians' willingness to prescribe. *Lancet.* 1994;343(8907):1209–1211.

33. Choudhry NK, Anderson GM, Laupacis A, Ross-Degnan D, Normand S-LT, Soumerai SB. Impact of adverse events on prescribing warfarin in patients with atrial fibrillation: matched pair analysis. *BMJ.* 2006;332(7534):141–145.

34. Aberegg SK, Haponik EF, Terry PB. Omission bias and decision making in pulmonary and critical care medicine. *Chest.* 2005;128(3):1497–1505.

35. Bergus GR, Chapman GB, Levy BT, Ely JW, Oppliger RA. Clinical diagnosis and the order of information. *Med Decis Mak.* 1998;18(4):412–417

36. Slevin ML, Stubbs L, Plant HJ, et al. Attitudes to chemotherapy: comparing views of patients with cancer with those of doctors, nurses, and general public. *BMJ (Clin Res Ed).* 1990;300(6737):1458–1460.

37. Christakis NA, Lamont EB. Extent and determinants of error in physicians' prognoses in terminally ill patients: prospective cohort study. *West J Med.* 2000;172(5):310–313.

38. Slovic P, Monahan J, MacGregor DG. Violence risk assessment and risk communication: the effects of using actual cases, providing instruction, and employing probability versus frequency formats. *Law Hum Behav.* 2000;24(3):271–296.

12

Shared Decision Making, Truth Telling, and the Recalcitrant Family

John D. Lantos

Many pediatricians have found themselves caring for a child who has a complex, chronic, life-limiting condition that will likely lead to death. The child is frequently hospitalized in the pediatric intensive care unit (PICU) with life-threatening complications such as sepsis or pneumonia.[1] The pediatricians feel that these treatments are not in the child's best interest. They think that cardiopulmonary resuscitation (CPR) would be futile and a do-not-resuscitate (DNR) order appropriate. They discuss this with the child's parents, but after a first meeting in which the subject was tentatively broached, the parents actively avoid further discussion. When the parents are cornered and a discussion is forced upon them, they make it clear that they do not want to make a decision. They say things like "Well, we don't really want to deal with that yet," "We will leave it in God's hands," or, sometimes, "Just do everything!"[2]

The parents don't explicitly say that they oppose a DNR order. Instead, they seem less concerned about the actual decision they face than they with their role in making plans for their child's future. Specifically, they don't want to be explicitly made accountable for the decision to withhold or withdraw life-sustaining treatment. When they are asked to authorize a DNR order, they refuse to do so. They don't want to participate in a process of shared decision making.

When parents respond to an invitation to participate in decision making by opting out, we should not necessarily conclude that they oppose decisions to limit medical interventions. Instead, we should ask whether something else entirely is going on. Specifically, we should consider the possibility that the process of shared decision making leads to parents feeling complicit in a plan that violates their values or their emotional needs. If that is the case, then there will be certain situations in which we should take a slightly different approach to shared decision making than the approach outlined in many of chapters in this volume. That slightly different approach involves a deliberate cultivation of ambiguity rather than precision in discussions about end-of-life decisions. To illustrate what I have in mind, I will use examples from fiction, poetry, and personal memoir.

The Ambiguous Conversation:
A Fictional Portrayal

Nobel Laureate Kenzaburo Oe's novel, *A Personal Matter*, is about a child born with a "brain hernia."[3] Though fictional, the book is deeply autobiographical. Oe himself had a son born with an encephalocele. The main character in the novel, a young man nicknamed "Bird," has a son with a similar brain lesion. The doctors want to operate. Bird doesn't want them to because he has been told that the child will have permanent, severe brain damage. Nevertheless, Bird feels tremendous guilt at the thought that, by not consenting to the operation, he would be authorizing his son's death.

Bird and the doctor have a conversation about withholding fluid and nutrition. The conversation is a marvel of ambiguity that allows both Bird and the doctor to come away thinking that the other made the decision to withhold treatment. The doctor approaches Bird at the baby's bedside. I recreate the conversation from the book, which is written with no attribution of particular statements to either Bird or the doctor.

"We'll have somebody from brain surgery examine the child in the next four or five days."
"Then—there will be an operation?"
"If the infant gets strong enough to withstand the surgery, yes." The doctor said, misinterpreting Bird's hesitation.
"Is there any possibility that the baby will grow up normally even if he is operated on? At the hospital where he was born yesterday, they said the most we could hope for even with surgery was a kind of vegetable existence."
"A vegetable—I don't know if I'd put it that way...." The doctor, without a direct reply to Bird's question, lapsed into silence.
"You don't want the baby to have an operation and recover, partially recover anyway?"
"Even with surgery, if the chances are very slight ... that he'll grow up to be a normal baby...."
"I suppose you realize that I can't take any direct steps to end the baby's life!"
"Of course not—"
"It's true that you're a young father—what, about my age." In a hushed voice that no one else on the ward could hear, he said, "Let's try regulating the baby's milk. We can even give him a sugar water substitute. We'll see how he does on that for a while...."
"Thank you," Bird said, with a dubious sigh.
"Don't mention it." (pp. 74–76)

Note a few things about this dialogue. First, Bird begins to signal his desire for the baby not to have surgery by asking an open-ended question: "Then there will be an operation?" He doesn't feel empowered to ask that the operation not take place. The doctor misinterprets the question as one about the baby's current physiological status, rather than about the ethical question of whether it is permissible to let the baby die. They then quibble about the proper way to describe the baby's long-term prognosis: "A vegetable existence?" Maybe. Bird then gets slightly more direct but still suggests that it is the doctor who might not want the baby to have an operation from which he can only "partially recover." The doctor finally gets it and clarifies that euthanasia is out of the question. Bird acknowledges. They tacitly agree on an ambiguous plan to withhold nutrition with the apparent goals of keeping the baby from getting strong enough to undergo surgery.

This dialogue is laced with double entendre, misunderstandings, hints, and evasions. At certain points, it is difficult to know which of the two characters is speaking. Nevertheless, they reach a decision. Here is the key point: they reached the decision in a way that neither of them feels individually responsible. Each could plausibly claim that it was the other who made the decision. It is a decision about which both are somewhat ashamed.

Would the discussion have gone better if the doctor had said, "We need to make a decision here. Do you want surgery or not? If not, then it would probably be appropriate to withdraw fluid and nutrition." If faced with that stark explicitness, Bird, in his deep ambivalence, likely would have rejected the idea out of hand and perhaps even have gotten mad at the doctor for proposing it.

Still, the discussion is problematic. Much was left unspoken. Much was assumed by both Bird and the doctor. Those assumptions could have been wildly erroneous. Such incomplete and ambiguous discussions seem inadequate compared to the approach that is customary in the United States today, an approach that insists on explicitly stated decisions that everyone explicitly endorses.

Oe suggests that, for some people facing some decisions at certain times, the stark truth may be too difficult to bear. Instead, he suggests, we may need to temper our expectations and goals. Maybe the best we can hope for is discussions like this one in which nobody appears to have explicitly made a decision but that nevertheless lead to an apparent consensus about a course of action.

Oe recognizes that people's emotional realities may be in conflict with their values or philosophical goals. Bird does not know what he wants. He is facing a dilemma and a set of choices that are wildly beyond anything he ever imagined. He is in no position to rationally consider the options and choose among them. He is trying to understand what it means to be a first-time father, what it means to face the prospect of raising a disabled baby, and what it would mean to be complicit in that baby's death. He doesn't want to be where he is. He is in pain.

Doctors, in such situations, offer messages that are themselves somewhat ambiguous. When we offer parents an explicit choice about CPR or a DNR order, even when we strongly believe that CPR would be futile, inappropriate, or even harmful, we send a deeply mixed message. Parents not unreasonably perceive the doctor's willingness to offer a choice as implicitly implying that either choice is reasonable. Many parents must think that if the doctors knew that CPR would not work, they would not be offering it. If they are offering, then it might work, and if that is the case, then the choice to try CPR can seem to be the most reasonable. Without it, the child will certainly die. With it, the child might not die. What is there to lose? The process of shared decision making in these circumstances is one that cannot even begin to address the decision that must be made until the emotional realities of the situation are acknowledged and their power respected.

What Sorts of Discussions Are the Most Respectful of Parents as Persons?

Most DNR policies mandate a discussion with parents, but they do not generally say what sort of discussion or how that discussion needs to go.

For example, the Kansas legislature recently passed a law stating that a DNR order cannot be instituted for an unemancipated minor unless at least one parent or legal guardian of the minor has been informed, orally and in writing, of the intent to institute the order. Either parent may refuse consent for a DNR or similar order, either orally or in writing. No DNR or similar order can be instituted if either parent does not agree to it.[4]

This law is an attempt to mandate transparency. But even this law allows ambiguity. It does not require parents to actually state their agreement to a DNR order. Instead, it only requires that they don't articulate a disagreement. In taking this approach, it endorses a concept proposed by Alex Kon, a concept that he called "informed non-dissent."[5] By this approach, the physician does not "ask." Instead, they inform the family that a decision has been made. If the surrogate does not object, they are presumed to have assented, and the plan of action may be implemented.

The nondissent approach leads to some key questions about the process of shared decision making. What, precisely, counts as a discussion about a DNR order? What, exactly, must be said to parents to believe that they have been sufficiently informed? Do we have to say, "We are going to write a DNR order for your baby"? Or would it be enough to say, "I am so sorry to tell you that your baby is dying, that we've tried everything, and that there is nothing more we can do. We are now going to remove the machines and let you hold your baby so that she can die comfortably in your arms." Or, "Our goal now is only to make sure that your baby doesn't suffer as she is dying. We will do everything we can to ensure that she has a peaceful death." If, after saying these things, the parents accept the plan, could we conclude that they have agreed to a DNR order? Neither laws nor hospital policies answer these questions.

Learning to Communicate Honestly but Indirectly

Burns and Truog write very insightfully about the need for good communication. They suggest that "ethics consults on 'futility' cases are far more commonly about breakdowns in communication and trust and far less often intractable disputes over the value assigned to medical facts."[6] Their view is that, often, patients and families do not truly disagree with doctors. Instead, they just don't understand and the reasons for their misunderstandings are because doctors are not good at "establishing a rapport, informing the family of the clinicians' opinions and answering any questions that the family may have."[7] This inadequate communication is, no doubt, common.

Sometimes, however, the communication breakdown is not from a family's lack of understanding. Instead, it is because families understand full well what is going on. They simply do not want to play the role that we have assigned to them, the role of final decision maker about the permissibility of withdrawing life support. To overcome this, the solution is not to have more explicitly honest discussions to clear up the facts. Instead, it might call for a different sort of communication, one that conveys the essential facts of the situation but in a way that is sensitive to the parents' need not to feel complicit, not to share in the decision, but, instead, to know what is going on and to be helped to accept it.

The inspiration for such indirect conveyance of difficult and frightening truths comes not from moral philosophers but, instead, from poetry. Emily Dickinson wrote a brilliant poem about truth telling. She wrote:

> Tell all the truth but tell it slant —
> Success in Circuit lies
> Too bright for our infirm Delight
> The Truth's superb surprise
>
> As Lightning to the Children eased
> With explanation kind
> The Truth must dazzle gradually
> Or every man be blind.

There are a few things to note about the Dickensonian approach. First, she opens the poem by saying that we should "tell all the truth." This is not an argument for partial truths, for dissembling, for hiding things. Second, she recognizes that sometimes the truth is terrifying. The image of a child's fear of lightning suggests how one might cower before a truth that is about something mind-boggling, something almost beyond our imagination. To calm our fears, Dickenson suggests, explanations may need to be circuitous. A blinding truth, she says, can be unkind.

What would a Dickensonian approach mean for shared decision making when the decision to be made is one that is deeply disturbing? Discussions in cases like the one earlier could take place without explicitly addressing the question of a DNR order or CPR. Instead, the doctor may say things like "We are doing all that we can but, sadly, it is not working," or "Given the situation, our only goal now is to keep Johnny comfortable." Families may respond to these cues with demands for specific treatments. Or they may respond with silent acknowledgment of the implicit truths that the doctor is conveying.

The doctor, in such cases, should accept nondissent as sufficient. There is no obligation to solicit agreement with a follow-up question such as "Is that OK with you?"

Accepting nondissent, rather than soliciting articulated agreement, can lead to better care of the patient and better psychological well-being for the family. We need to get better at conversations that tell the truth slant, that convey a message, that offer an opportunity for dissent, but that don't demand assent. Such conversations allow parents an escape from an intolerable feeling of complicity.

Tragic Choices

The moral force behind this approach comes from the recognition that a decision to allow a child to die is a tragic choice. Both options are irredeemably bad—to continue painful and futile treatments or to agree to withdraw life support and let one's baby die. When faced with a tragic choice, good people necessarily and inevitably feel ambivalent.[8] People may recognize that their loved one is dying, realize the CPR will be futile, but still not wish to be complicit in "giving up" on a loved one or endorsing the withdrawal of treatment.[9] In such situations, people clearly want something but they also—and equally passionately—do not want to take individual moral responsibility for the decision. Their unacknowledged desire becomes a shameful secret.

A beautiful description of this appears in a book by Alan Shapiro about his sister Beth's death. Beth was dying of cancer. The family sat at her bedside for days, waiting for her to die. He makes the following striking confession: "We were tired of seeing her languish, tired of the degradation we were helpless to do anything about. We were tired of our helplessness and guilty for being tired. That we were all impatient to go home was our unspoken wish, our dirty secret"[10] (p. 10).

Shapiro goes on, "We wished for any sort of illusory refuge, or palatable lie that might blunt what we were helpless not to feel."[10] When people are helpless not to feel something that they do not want to feel, they may seek ambiguity rather than accountability, and may prefer deniability to responsibility.[11] They may hint at their understanding and their wishes but shrink back from an explicit acknowledgment of what they truly want. Explicitness might work against empowerment here and become cruel or coercive.

In such circumstances, the best decisions, from the perspective of the participants, may be those in which it is not clear who really made the decision or who even understood that a decision was being made at a certain point. This allows them to deny any complicity in the actions that follow. Each is able to believe—or believe enough—that someone else made the decision.

Practical Implications

This brief inquiry suggests that the moral psychology of tragic choices is quite different from what has been imagined by many leading bioethicists. Bioethicists emphasize the importance of individual choice and autonomy. The moral psychologists describe processes by which individuals avoid choice and submerge their autonomy into a collective will.

This process currently occurs in many cases. Doctors, patients, ethicists, and family members often invoke "futility," talk of "what Dad would have wanted," or request that we "let nature take its course." In so doing, they are not trying to exercise their own will. Instead, they are trying to submerge their own will so that they can become passive agents of a larger, seemingly inexorable force.

This approach recognizes that different people come to the truth in different ways. This approach was encapsulated by Bonhoeffer, who wrote, "the truth is not a quantity that in itself is constant, but is as alive as life itself. Where it looses itself from life and from the relationship to the concrete other person, where the 'truth is told' without observing to whom I say it, there it has only the appearance but not the essence of truth."[12]

Telling the truth slant requires imagination sensitivity to the parents' nonverbal cues. Those cues reveal their values and preferences as much as their verbal utterances. The goal of shared decision making can only be reached if doctors not only listen very carefully to what parents are saying but also listen to what they are not saying but are nevertheless trying hard to communicate. Sometimes they may be saying that there are things that they want but prefer not to discuss or decisions that they endorse but would prefer not to affirm.

References

1. Paris JJ, Crone RK, Reardon F. Physicians' refusal of requested treatment. *N Engl J Med.* 1989;322:1012–1014.
2. Miller RB. *Children, Ethics, and Modern Medicine.* Bloomington: University of Indiana Press; 2003:120–144.
3. Oe K. *A Personal Matter.* New York: Grove Press; 1994.
4. http://www.kslegislature.org/li/b2017_18/measures/documents/summary_sb_85_2017.pdf. Accessed September 28, 2017.
5. Kon AA. Informed non-dissent: a better option than slow codes when families cannot bear to say "Let her die." *Am J Bioeth.* 2011;11:22–23.
6. Burns JP, Truog RD. Futility. A concept in evolution. *Chest.* 2007;132:1987–1993.
7. Sibbald R, Downar J, Hawryluck L. Perceptions of "futile care" among caregivers in intensive care units. *CMAJ.* 2007;177:1201–1208.
8. Dostoevsky F. *The Brothers Karamazov.* New York: Signet; 1962.
9. Azoulay E, Pochard F, Chevret S, et al. Half the family members of intensive care unit patients do not want to share in the decision-making process: a study in 78 French intensive care units. *Crit Care Med.* 2004;32:1832–1838.
10. Shapiro A. *Vigil.* Chicago: University of Chicago; 1997:82.
11. Montello MM, Lantos JD. The Karamazov complex: Dostoevsky and DNR orders. *Perspect Biol Med.* 2002;45:190–199.
12. Moberly J. *The Virtue of Bonhoeffer's Ethics. A Study of Dietrich Bonhoeffer's Ethics in Relation to Virtue Ethics.* Eugene, OR: Pickwick Publications; 2013:158.

Index